HOW OUR ANCESTORS DIED

A Guide for Family Historians

SIMON WILLS

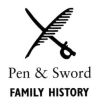

Pen & Sword
FAMILY HISTORY

First published in Great Britain in 2013 by
PEN AND SWORD FAMILY HISTORY
an imprint of
Pen & Sword Books Ltd
47 Church Street
Barnsley
South Yorkshire
S70 2AS

ISBN 978 1 78159 038 6

Typeset in 10pt Palatino by Mac Style, Driffield, East Yorkshire
Printed and bound in the UK by CPI Group (UK) Ltd, Croydon, CR0 4YY

Pen & Sword Books Ltd incorporates the Imprints of Pen & Sword
Aviation, Pen & Sword Family History, Pen & Sword Maritime, Pen
& Sword Military, Pen & Sword Discovery, Wharncliffe Local History,
Wharncliffe True Crime, Wharncliffe Transport, Pen & Sword Select,
Pen & Sword Military Classics, Leo Cooper, The Praetorian Press,
Remember When, Seaforth Publishing and Frontline Publishing.

For a complete list of Pen & Sword titles please contact
PEN & SWORD BOOKS LIMITED
47 Church Street, Barnsley, South Yorkshire, S70 2AS, England
E-mail: enquiries@pen-and-sword.co.uk
Website: www.pen-and-sword.co.uk

CONTENTS

Preface vi

Chapter 1   Investigation, Diagnosis, and Treatment of Disease . . 1

Chapter 2   Finding a Cause of Death 17

Chapter 3   Accidents and Disasters 30

Chapter 4   Alcohol and Alcoholism 40

Chapter 5   Cancer 47

Chapter 6   Chest Conditions 53

Chapter 7   Children, Babies, and Infection 61

Chapter 8   Cholera 70

Chapter 9   Diet and Starvation 77

Chapter 10 Dysentery and Bowel Infections 86

Chapter 11 Epilepsy and Strokes 94

Chapter 12 Execution and Murder 99

Chapter 13 Heart Conditions 109

Chapter 14 Influenza 116

Chapter 15 Mental Illness and Suicide 119

Chapter 16 Opium Addiction 131

Chapter 17 Plague 138

Chapter 18 Pregnancy and Childbirth 143

Chapter 19 Scurvy 150

Chapter 20 Smallpox 157

Chapter 21 Tropical Infections 164

Chapter 22 Tuberculosis 169

Chapter 23 Typhus 176

Chapter 24 Venereal Diseases 183

Chapter 25 War 190

Chapter 26 Wounds 196

Chapter 27 Places to Visit 203

Bibliography 209

Index 210

To Mike, Annie, Branty, Caf, Kate, and Nick – good friends; and the modern doctors and nurses that we should all be grateful for.

PREFACE

An ancestor's death can often tell you something about their life, and may turn out to be one of the most thought-provoking things that you know about them. For the past 400 years, my ancestors have all come from the same small town and yet tracing their deaths has revealed the surprising breadths of their wanderings – a nineteenth-century trader died of cholera in Poland, another of yellow fever in Barbados, and one man died of scurvy in Sri Lanka in the eighteenth century. Their deaths also told me about the hardships they suffered in life – I have an ancestor with dementia who was murdered in a workhouse, an alcoholic stepmother who died of a stroke at a young age, and two fishermen who drowned at sea, one of whom had to work well into his seventies because he couldn't afford to stop working.

The circumstances of an ancestor's death may also help you understand more about the lives of the family that was left behind – the husband forced to re-marry after the death of his wife so that someone would look after his children; the wife thrown into poverty after the death of her husband; the woman who loses her husband to enemy action and then sees her son go off to war as well; the man who has to continue working in the same mine in which his brother was killed.

A book of this size could never hope to cover all possible causes of death, but I have focused on those that commonly or uniquely affected our ancestors. I've also tried to show how some medical conditions offer significant insight into historical attitudes to health and disease, explained how the dying were likely to be treated, and drawn attention to causes of death that were linked to particular occupations or roles. I have indicated alternative names for medical conditions throughout the book to help you make sense of what doctors wrote, and these are all included in the index for easy reference. I have also tried to illustrate the text with contemporary accounts of deaths that should offer some appreciation of our ancestors' experiences, although note that I have often modernised spellings and punctuation to make these more readable.

My most immediate feeling on finishing this book was one of relief. Not so much because I had completed such a big task, but because I fully realised what a trial life must have been for our ancestors. With so many threats to life as part of everyday existence, it's a wonder that anyone survived into old age at all.

We've come a long way.

Smallpox, one of the greatest killers of all time, has been eradicated, and diseases such as plague and cholera that once invaded our shores periodically to destroy communities no longer do so. Other diseases formerly endemic to Britain such as malaria, typhus, and diphtheria are no longer a threat, and we no longer lose members of our families to scurvy, famine, or armed rebellion.

The chances of our babies and children dying, or of pregnant women not surviving labour, are enormously reduced – even compared to a hundred years ago. Vaccines mean that many diseases of childhood such as measles or whooping cough have been kept at bay, and antibiotics now quickly treat infections that blighted or destroyed our ancestors' lives such as scarlet fever and venereal disease. In our modern world we do not worry that a mere wound will become infected and kill us or cause us to lose a limb, and if we have to have surgery we know that our chances of surviving it are the best they have ever been. Despite silly extremes of 'health and safety' being the butt of much ironic humour these days, a more safety conscious society now means that we have a much greater chance of surviving a simple journey or a day at work than our ancestors.

Many of the medical problems discussed in this book still confront us but to a very much lesser extent than in the past: we still have bowel infections in Britain, for example, but on a smaller scale than in the past, and modern medicines make it unlikely that we will die from them. Experts tell us that influenza keeps threatening to break out in lethally epic proportions, as it has done in the past, but mercifully at the time of writing has not done so recently. TB still haunts us, but on nothing like the scale of the past.

In other cases, we still have some way to go. Although cancer is not the automatic death sentence it was in Victorian times, especially if caught early, lots of people still die from it in our modern world. However, many others are now cured or have their lives extended significantly by contemporary treatments. Heart disease, strokes, and mental illness still sadly afflict many people, but these days we can do more to treat and support those affected than we ever could before. Preventive healthcare also means we can now go some way towards averting many modern medical conditions too.

We still sometimes worry about the behaviour of drunken people in our communities today, but this is a pale reflection of the widespread public anarchy caused by alcohol in the eighteenth century. Even those convicted of the most serious crimes need no longer fear the hangman's noose or the executioner's axe. And whilst accidents still happen, and so do wars, the numbers of British citizens affected are far fewer than in earlier centuries.

So whilst this book deals with a (literally) morbid subject, it does carry a positive message for us in the modern world: we've never had it so good in terms of our chances of living a long and healthy life. Our ancestors were very much less fortunate.

Chapter 1

INVESTIGATION, DIAGNOSIS, AND TREATMENT OF DISEASE

Not all deaths are caused by disease, but a major proportion of this book is devoted to medical conditions that killed our ancestors, so it's appropriate to begin with a chapter devoted to disease and healthcare.

These days we have great freedom to learn about illness for ourselves if we want to. We can read the same books and websites as our doctors, and even look at original clinical research. But it wasn't that long ago that medical knowledge was virtually the sole province of doctors who guarded it jealousy. Paradoxically, despite this 'protectionism' a high proportion of what the medical profession thought they knew about disease before the late Victorian era was simply wrong.

Identifying Diseases

Apart from finding a cause of death in the first place (see Chapter 2), a significant problem for anyone interested in investigating the diseases that affected our forebears is the accuracy of diagnoses in former times. It's very clear that medical terms could often be used quite loosely. Some diseases have very characteristic or unique symptoms and so diagnosis is more likely to be accurate: smallpox, for example. However, in other circumstances a diagnosis might cover a multitude of ills. The man or woman in the seventeenth century who died of 'griping in the guts' died of what? Appendicitis? A peptic ulcer? An intestinal infection? Bowel cancer?

A diagnosis might cover a range of possibilities and perhaps the most notorious of these is the word 'fever', which indicates an infection but what kind? The circumstances might give you clues, but without more detail one can only speculate. Similarly, the diagnosis of 'dropsy' meant that someone had a build-up of fluid in the body, but it might have been by a variety of means – heart failure or kidney disease being two principal contenders.

You should also note that some words with quite precise meanings these days might have been more mutable in the past. In our modern world the diagnosis of 'pleurisy' means a quite particular disease of the lungs, but reading accounts of 'pleurisy' in the past it seems as if it was sometimes used to refer to all sorts of chest complaints.

Even when there was an outbreak of an infectious disease in a community, chroniclers of the time may provide such limited detail that it is not possible to identify it reliably. In the sixteenth and late fifteenth centuries, for example, Britain was periodically ravaged by 'the sweating sickness'. There were outbreaks in 1485, 1502, 1507, 1517, 1528, and 1551. However, it is described so scantily in contemporary sources that even now we are not sure what disease this was. The fever, joint ache and exhaustion suggest these may have been a series of severe influenza epidemics, but we will probably never know for sure. And it seems that the characteristics of an epidemic disease may change according to the strain of infectious micro-organism – so the flu epidemic of 1918 killed many, many more people than that of 1889 or 1957.

What Killed Our Ancestors?

Table 1 on the page opposite compares the top ten leading causes of death in random years chosen from the last five centuries. Of course it's not really fair to make direct comparisons between these eras because, as noted above, the identification and classification of diseases has varied so much over the centuries. As time has progressed, diagnosis has become more accurate.

However, a general comparison is interesting. Infections such as TB, smallpox, 'fever', plague, typhus, and even whooping cough dominate the era before antibiotics and vaccines. The prevalence of 'convulsions' as a cause of death probably reflects the high mortality for infants and newborn babies from infections in earlier times because fever in the very young may cause them to fit. Meningitis is another potential cause of fitting. Many of the cases of 'asthma' and 'bronchitis' in former times are probably what we would now call 'chest infections', although some may have been lung cancer.

Heart disease, cancer, and strokes only became more common in the twentieth century when people began to live long enough to develop these diseases which are more likely as people reach their late middle age. Similarly, dementia is largely a disease of the late twentieth century onwards when a high proportion of the population began to live beyond 75 years of age. 'Old age' features as a common cause of death in the seventeenth, eighteenth, and nineteenth centuries and probably reflects

Table 1: Top ten commonest causes of death for the years given, over the last five centuries.

1660s (London)	1750s (London)	1838 (England and Wales)	1930 (England and Wales)	2010 (England and Wales)
Plague	Convulsions	Tuberculosis	Heart disease	Heart attack
Tuberculosis	Tuberculosis	Old age	Stroke	Stroke
Fever	Fever of various kinds	Convulsions	Tuberculosis	Lung cancer
Miscarriage, stillbirth, newborn baby	Smallpox	Typhus	Bronchitis	Other long-term lung diseases
Griping in the guts	Old age	Pneumonia	Cancer of gut and liver	Influenza and pneumonia
Convulsions	Teeth	Smallpox	Pneumonia	Dementia
Teeth and worms	Dropsy	Debility	Babies at or near birth	Breast cancer
Aged and bedridden	Miscarriage, stillbirth	Dropsy	Senile dementia	Prostate cancer
Dropsy	Asthma and coughs	Violence and accidents	Kidney and bladder disease	Urinary diseases
Smallpox	Violence and accidents	Whooping cough	Accidents	Heart failure

(Sources: The data for the ten years of the 1660s and 1750s are from the *Yearly Bills of Mortality* for London; data for 1838 is derived from the second *Annual Report of the Registrar-general of Births, Deaths, and Marriages*; and 1930 and 2010 data are taken from the Office of National Statistics website www.statistics.gov.uk)

a combination of all these medical conditions, but in former times many of the diseases of older adults were not diagnosed or even medically recognised.

It is a little alarming to see that violence and accidents feature in the top ten only comparatively recently. However, technological developments in transport and safer working practices now mean that travel and the workplace are a lot safer than in previous centuries.

Life Expectancy

In the past, the average inhabitant of the British Isles had very little money, and many had insufficient food, lacked clean water, and had inadequate shelter. In addition to poor sanitation and an increased likelihood of malnutrition, our forebears were assaulted by many more diseases that could cause life-threatening illness at an early age – particularly infections. This meant that a high proportion of babies and infants died, resulting in a considerably lower average life expectancy for the population. Thus, the average life expectancy of a newborn child in the sixteenth century was only in the mid-thirties, and it did not reach 40 until about 1800. Even in 1901 the average lifespan for a newborn boy stood at only 45 years of age, and for girls this was 49 years. The twentieth century, however, saw enormous social and technological strides and so by 2010 the average life expectancy at birth for a newborn baby boy was 78.5 years of age, and 82.4 years for a girl. A staggering improvement in just over a hundred years.

Why do we now live longer? There are many reasons. Sanitation was an important early step. It meant that sewage was separated from what our ancestors drank so there was clean drinking water. This has made typhoid, cholera, and dysentery diseases of the past in this country. Vaccination was another vital advance that started in the nineteenth century. It has drastically reduced the huge mortality due to infections such as smallpox, tuberculosis, and diphtheria. Improved national prosperity and social welfare meant that even the poorest people in society began to experience significantly improved incomes in the twentieth century. More money allowed people to buy enough food, and to afford accommodation offering greater personal space and therefore less overcrowding. In the past, malnutrition increased people's susceptibility to disease, and overcrowding allowed infectious diseases like typhus to spread quickly. Finally, many medical advances have been revolutionary. There are too many to identify them all here, but important changes include the discovery of antibiotics, the proper training of doctors along scientific lines, the improved ability to diagnose disease early using imaging machines and blood analysis, and the use of preventive healthcare to encourage healthy lifestyles and disease awareness.

Theories of Disease

Before science began to reveal the true causes, doctors had some very odd beliefs about the origins of disease. These notions affected their whole approach to the patient and to treatment for centuries.

The Greek philosophers in the fifth century BCE built up theories describing our physical world. According to these concepts, all matter on our planet was composed of four principal 'elements' – fire, air, water, and earth – and each of these elements were described by four 'qualities' – dry, hot, wet, and cold. The qualities worked in pairs so the element 'fire' was dry and hot, whereas 'water' was wet and cold, and so on.

The work of Hippocrates and associated classical doctors added a medical layer to this pattern of four elements and qualities. Four 'humours' were said to enjoy a natural balance in the human body and when that balance was disrupted, then disease resulted. These four humours were blood, phlegm, black bile (melancholy), and yellow bile (choler), and later came to be associated with four corresponding human 'temperaments' – sanguine, phlegmatic, melancholic, and choleric respectively. In time, doctors came to believe that all of these factors were affected differently by the four 'seasons', and also interplayed with the twelve 'signs of the Zodiac'.

The endlessly complicated interplay between these four elements, qualities, humours, temperaments, and seasons was what caused disease, but a successful understanding of the imbalance also yielded clues to the treatment that would succeed. It is all quite bizarre to us in the modern world, but this strangely complex and totally unfounded theory persisted in various forms into the nineteenth century. Cynically, its complexity might be seen as a way to keep disease a mystery and thus allow doctors to preserve their authority, but perhaps more prosaically there was simply nothing else to take its place.

However, despite the dominance of this so-called humoural theory, there were other forces at work that doctors and patients alike believed could cause disease. Amongst these, mystical forces came to the fore: in medieval times, witchcraft was believed to cause disease, and astrology or the stars were said to affect health. Lunacy, for example, was a derangement caused by the goddess of the moon herself, Luna. There were also religious aspects of disease – a person with epilepsy might be said to be possessed by a devil, and those who died very suddenly were struck down by 'visitation of God'. Moral laxity was frequently cited as the cause of all sorts of diseases from scurvy to tuberculosis, because many people believed well into the nineteenth century that God singled out sinful people for punishment with nasty diseases.

From the seventeenth century onwards, doctors gradually began to understand more about how the body worked, but lack of basic scientific knowledge always hindered significant advances. In very general terms, until the mid to late nineteenth century, most disease was thought to be caused by one of three things – environment, behaviour, or diet – and these causes were sometimes related back to their potential effects upon the humours. Medical men – and they were men alone until the twentieth century – found it difficult to imagine any causes beyond these basic three. So, when it came to environmental causes, for example, foul-smelling air or miasma was believed to precipitate diseases such as cholera, malaria, and dysentery. And some doctors spent many hours plotting weather patterns and trying to tie them to particular diseases, or speculating on climatic conditions that would bring forth epidemics.

Human behaviour was a natural place, perhaps, to begin looking for a cause of disease. Regrettably, though, doctors sometimes allowed themselves to become entangled in the prevailing moral messages of the day. This meant that in Victorian society, for example, a doctor visiting your unfortunate ancestor suffering from dementia, tuberculosis, or mental illness might conclude that they were ill because they had masturbated too much. Diet was also the source of some odd ideas about the causation of disease – rashes might be caused by eating 'cold' vegetables such as cucumbers, whilst fruits and vegetables that produced flatulence had to be avoided by those with asthma.

We now know that most diseases are caused by micro-organisms, genetics, lifestyle (e.g. diet), immune reactions, and chemicals (e.g. smoking). Although the basis of many of these discoveries were laid in the nineteenth century, the full realisation of their role in causing disease – and the discovery of the most appropriate methods of treatment – had to await the twentieth century.

Treatments

The further back one travels in time, the worse the situation becomes in terms of treatment for our unfortunate ancestors. In medieval times, for example, people were peddled amulets or charms, and given magical words to say, or even wear, to promote healing.

Before the twentieth century there was virtually no application of what might be termed 'the scientific method' when it came to selecting and identifying any medical treatment. These days we rely on clinical trials to show if a treatment works. Crudely, this means that large numbers of patients given one treatment for a disease are compared to patients given no treatment (or a different one). However, in the past doctors generally relied on the same old treatments that classical authors had advocated for centuries, the latest fad that had been reported in the medical press, or they jumped upon some chance 'discovery' of their own that seemed to work in one patient. Hindsight is a wonderful thing, but it's clear that the best they could offer most patients was of very limited value indeed; a lot of it probably made, at best, no difference, whilst some of their treatments were actually detrimental.

Nonetheless, many of our ancestors' doctors and surgeons were as passionate as their modern counterparts concerning the well-being of their patients: they did the best that they could with the tools and knowledge at their disposal. But at the other extreme there were less scrupulous individuals who realised that human illness was a means to make a living from a credulous and desperate clientele. There were also a great number of 'fad' treatments that came and went just as they do today, such as strange diets, mysterious foreign 'medicines', spa waters, magnetism, electricity, fumigation, and many more.

All in all, the prospect of medical attention did not fill many of our ancestors with much hope – it was just the only hope they had other than the Church – and so the more realistic put little faith in what doctors had

A nineteenth-century advertisement for leeches that doctors used for bloodletting. The Hambro Speckled and the Officinal Green were species of medicinal leech.

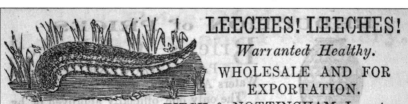

to offer. The essayist Joseph Addison remarked in the early eighteenth century that 'when a nation abounds in physicians it grows thin of people'.

Blood, Bowels, and Blisters

Until the late nineteenth century, becoming a doctor meant largely accepting certain practices and concepts blindly 'on faith', because everyone else did. The concept of having 'proof' that a treatment worked, was an alien one. No areas of medical practice reflect this better than the three most universally popular treatments that doctors dished out unquestioningly until the late nineteenth century, simply because their illustrious predecessors had.

Bleeding the patient, or 'bloodletting', is an excellent example of this, as it was used for almost any condition imaginable and was accepted by doctor and patient alike for centuries. Diseases were thought to produce toxins that disrupted the body's natural balance and thus they needed to be released from the body. Bloodletting was thought to achieve this by purifying the blood. The practice of bleeding the patient meant the doctor using small slug-like animals called leeches that sucked the blood out, or using a sharp blade or lancet to open a patient's a vein so that they bled into a bowl. This treatment would simply have weakened the already ill patient by causing anaemia and disrupting the body's fluid balance, and in many cases probably hastened their end.

Similarly, laxatives were used in many forms to purify the bowel. It is not an exaggeration to say that our ancestors' doctors were obsessed with the human bowel. Its 'dirty' contents were often thought of as the seat of disease even for conditions that had no obvious connection with the intestines such as asthma. Various plant extracts were used for this purpose – including senna, cascara, and rhubarb – and they were often referred to as purgatives or cathartics. Solutions poured into the bowel as enemas (or clysters) were employed for similar purposes. Emetics were also used very commonly to tackle the bowel from the other end by making the patient vomit. The commonest medicine used for this was a plant called ipecacuanha. Doctors persisted with their addiction to these treatments even if the patient already had profuse diarrhoea or vomiting because of their illness. So whether it was cholera or a stroke the patient's bowels were forced open at both ends. This must have frequently led to the patient becoming dehydrated – particularly if they already had diarrhoea and vomiting – and so probably hastened the end for many.

Apart from blood and bowel, our unfortunate ancestors' doctors' third fixation was with the human skin. Yet again, this passion persevered for centuries irrespective of whether there was any obvious connection between the skin and the medical condition concerned. In particular, doctors were enthusiastic about irritating the skin to allow disease-causing poisons to escape the body via this route. Threads sewn under the surface of the skin known as 'setons' helped to bring forth pus and offer the disease an escape route from the body. Doctors also employed agents such as caustic potash, acids, or Cantharides (an insect also known as 'Spanish fly') to cause open sores or blistering. Irritant plasters were often applied to the abdomen to redden the skin without blistering, and mustard plasters or 'sinapisms' were common. Perhaps the strangest of all was the technique known as 'cupping', whereby a cup was heated and applied to the skin so that it drew up a mound of skin by suction as the air inside the cup cooled. Sometimes this was combined with bloodletting.

Medicines

The power of prayer has been invoked when faced with serious illness since the dawn of Christianity. In medieval times monasteries and convents offered physical treatments as well as heavenly intervention, and were important sources of healthcare advice and medication in a community. Yet there have been some curious religious twists to the story of human treatment of disease. The Doctrine of Signatures, for example, arose in the sixteenth century, and its advocates suggested that God left little clues to plants that may be of benefit to healing humankind. These were the endorsement or signature of the Almighty on the power of the potential cure. For example, walnuts look like little skulls with a brain inside so they were used to treat disorders of the head such as mental illness.

Plants (or 'vegetable' cures) were the principal early medicines used to treat human illness, and a glance through any pre-twentieth-century medical book throws light on some very imaginative uses and intriguing concoctions. In *The English Physician (Enlarged)* (1666), Nicholas Culpepper writes about the cornflower:

> As they are naturally cold, dry, and binding, so they are under the dominion of Saturn. The powder or dried leaves of the blue-bottle, or corn-flower, is given with good success to those that are bruised by a fall, or have broken a vein inwardly, and void much blood at the mouth; being taken in the water of plantain, horse-tail, or the greater comfrey, it is a remedy against the poison of the scorpion, and resisteth all venoms and poisons. The seed or leaves taken in wine, is very good against the

plague, and all infectious diseases, and is very good in pestilential fevers. The juice put into fresh or green wounds, doth quickly solder up the lips of them together, and is very effectual to heal all ulcers and sores in the mouth. The juice dropped into the eyes takes away the heat and inflammation of them. The distilled water of this herb, hath the same properties, and may be used for the effects aforesaid.

Charming though Culpepper's style of writing is, most of what he says is simply nonsense. His, and other medical writers', instructions were based on many previous generations of opinions, bad ideas, and misconceptions. The ideas of ancient writers such Galen, Hippocrates, and other worthies were simply accepted de facto from one generation to the next, with each era adding its own accretions.

Medicines were also derived from animals. An eighteenth-century list of medicinal treatments might include sea horses (*hippocampus*), woodlice (*millepedes*), reindeer hooves (*ungula alces*), ivory (*ebur*), musk (*moschus*), goat's blood (*sanguis hirci*), mummified human remains from Egypt (*mumia*), and honey (*mel*). Contemporary physician John Hill has this to say on the subject of woodlice in his *History of the Materia Medica* (1751):

> We sometimes give the animals dry'd and reduced to powder, but in this state they lose the greater part of their virtues. The best way of taking them is the swallowing them alive; this is very easily and conveniently done for they naturally roll themselves up on being touch'd, and thus form a sort of smooth pill, which easily slips down the throat...
>
> Woodlice ... are aperient [laxative], attenuant [thin the blood], and detergent; they dissolve viscous humours, are good in all obstructions of the viscera, and have even been celebrated by some writers as a remedy for the [kidney] stone ... They are often found to be of service in asthma, and great good has been sometimes done by a long course of them in disorders of the eyes.

Apart from living sources certain chemicals, metals, or rocks were also used medicinally. Usually termed 'minerals' or 'fossils', they included things such as arsenic, coral, slate, amethyst, antimony, copper, vitriol (sulphuric acid), and nitre (potassium nitrate).

Some treatments were used for centuries because belief in them was so strong. One of the most notable examples is mercury: this silvery liquid metal has fascinated investigators of all kinds down the ages. Surely this most unique of substances must have special properties? As a metal it was known as 'quicksilver' and the rocks containing it 'cinnabar'. It was employed most commonly in the form of a solid compound called calomel, and was used to treat virtually everything: syphilis, TB, cholera, dysentery, yellow fever, gout, rheumatism, scurvy, worms, and many others. It continued to be a treatment for syphilis well into the twentieth century.

Physicians knew that mercury was dangerous too. The Roman poet Virgil famously remarked in the first century BCE that 'the medicine increases the disease', and this was particularly true of mercury. It is, however, a good example of how our ancestors' doctors knew something about side effects – the bad aspects of a medicine – as well as the alleged good sides, as evidenced by John Hill in his *History of the Materia Medica* (1751):

> We are not however to imagine that too free a use of so powerful a medicine as quicksilver, whether internally or externally, can be always without danger. We find that the unhappy creatures who work in the [cinnabar] mines seldom live more than three or four years and then die in most miserable conditions, and the people who work it in any other manner in abundance and for a constancy, are as certain of mischief from it. Palsies and tremblings of the limbs always attend this, and we have had abundant experience from the common mercurial unguents [ointments], and from the method of taking it internally, that when proper care has not been taken the nerves have been frequently terribly hurt by it, the humours colliquated [became fluid], and beside common symptoms of a ptyalism [drooling], ulcers of the mouth and throat, and diarrhoea of the most dangerous kind have been brought on.

Mercury was fascinating and everyone was keen to find new medical uses for it despite the fact that there is little evidence that it worked. At the other extreme, doctors with proof of an effective treatment often struggled to be heard. Before the twentieth century, medical views about disease management were more likely to be taken up because of the social or political influence of the author, rather than the scientific validity of his claims. For years, for example, James Lind's evidence showing that citrus juice cured scurvy was ignored – despite his careful scientific method in the world's first clinical trial – in favour of ridiculous,

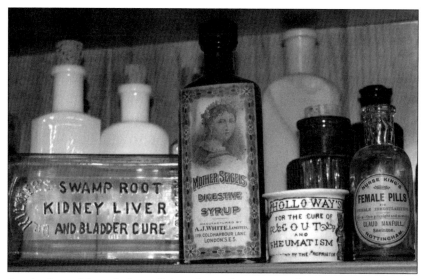

A selection of branded medicines from the nineteenth and early twentieth centuries.

foundless treatments preferred by the Admiralty's more influential doctors. John Snow, who first demonstrated that cholera was caused by contaminated water, and Edward Jenner, who provided the evidence that a vaccine could be used to prevent smallpox, were similarly overlooked initially because their influence was insignificant. The quality of their evidence was immaterial: they simply didn't have the ears of the powerful. Sadly this means in each case that many thousands of our ancestors died in the interim.

When our ancestors were ill they were, therefore, vulnerable to being exploited by people peddling all sorts of nonsense as medicines – from their doctor to a roadside seller. Before the eighteenth century, branded medicines of this type were often known as nostrums (from *nostrum remedium*, 'our remedy' in Latin), but they gradually came to be known as 'patent medicines'. They had names that extolled their curative powers and often promoted the originator – Dr Kilmer's Swamp Root Kidney, Liver and Bladder Cure; Mother Seigel's Digestive Syrup; Holloway's Universal Family Ointment; Daffy's Elixir of Health, and so on.

These medicines were commonly purported to contain exotic ingredients, and were often advertised as being treatments for a bewildering array of unrelated medical conditions. Holloway's Ointment, for instance, was sold for the cure of gout and rheumatism, inveterate ulcers, indolent tumours, burns, scrofula, insect bites, chilblains, boils, sore breasts, sore heads, bad legs 'etcetera'. Adverts haled these medicines as sensational breakthroughs with thousands of satisfied customers. What they really contained is open to much doubt; they were frequently liquid medicines so in many cases they were probably little more than pleasantly flavoured, coloured water. Yet people bought them in droves. Some of them were actually dangerous – Mrs Winslow's Soothing Syrup was designed to put infants to sleep, but contained large amounts of morphine and killed some children.

In his *Citizen of the World* (1765), Oliver Goldsmith explained with notable sarcasm that:

> Whatever may be the merits of the English in other sciences, they are peculiarly excellent in the art of healing. There is scarcely a disorder incident to humanity against which our advertising doctors are not possessed with a most infallible antidote. The professors of other arts confess the inevitable intricacy of things, talk with doubt, and decide with hesitation; but doubting is entirely unknown in medicine. The advertising professors here delight in cases of difficulty: be the disorder never so desperate or radical, you will find numbers in every street who, by levelling a pill at the part affected, promise a certain cure.

However, the medical profession were equally guilty of being gullible, or maybe naive. They frequently latched onto an allegedly new 'cure' proposed by a colleague and bandied it about in their professional publications. One reads endless examples in eighteenth and nineteenth-century medical books that 'Dr X from such-and-such reports favourably on the use of A to treat B'. No one thought to ask for proof. Worse than this, in many ways, were the doctors who developed 'secret cures' with ingredients they would not disclose but with 'many sworn affidavits as to the success of this treatment'.

A more understandable quirk of the medical profession in former times was to take a new medicine that did work, and try it out for lots of other diseases. Unfortunately, the result was usually that medicines with proven value for one medical condition were employed incessantly for many other diseases where they had no value. A good example here is quinine, which cured malaria so it was tried for any other condition with a fever. It didn't work, but that didn't stop doctors using it. The invaluable drug opium similarly was subject to a myriad of inappropriate uses.

All in all, before 1900, there were very few medicines taken by mouth that had any proven worth. Apart from an endless list of laxatives, digitalis was successfully used to treat heart failure, opium to treat pain, valerian for insomnia, quinine for malaria, and the new drug aspirin for pain and fever but there wasn't much else that we would value today. Most of it simply didn't work; a lot of it in the wrong hands was potentially rather dangerous.

A notable feature of medicines as the nineteenth century progressed was that the active ingredient of some medicinally active plants was isolated and then provided in pure form. Thus quinine was derived from Peruvian bark and found to be the chemical that cured and prevented malaria, and morphine was isolated from opium. Similarly, salicylates were discovered to be the active anti-inflammatory ingredient in willow bark and meadowsweet. However, here researchers went a step further: salicylates could be easily modified in the laboratory to produce acetyl-salicylic acid or aspirin and this was marketed as a new medicine in 1899. It was one of the first entirely synthetic 'chemicals' based on a plant molecule to be used medicinally. The modern pharmaceutical industry had begun, and in the twentieth century it would soon move away from plant sources to the laboratory for its inspiration.

The Caring Professions

Who were the professionals who might minister to your dying ancestor? In medieval times the Church had an important role to play, with many people visiting a monastery or convent for medical advice and treatment. The Church continued to have a role in burying the dead, and in ministering to the spiritual needs of the dying and bereaved, but

A gathering of physicians in the early years of the nineteenth century.

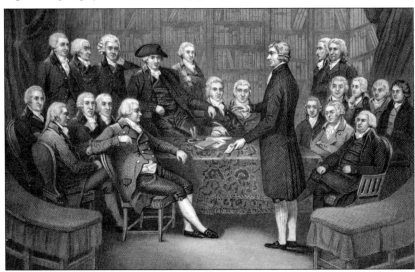

its involvement in healthcare waned as more specialist practitioners evolved.

Until the eighteenth century the forerunners of our modern doctors fulfilled a variety of separate roles and were not clearly identifiable as one profession. Surgeons undertook operations, but there were few specialists until the late nineteenth century so many of them took on everything from bowel surgery to amputations. They were also known as chirurgeons, especially if they were attached to the army or navy which employed a great many. Physicians diagnosed illness and treated it without surgery, using their knowledge of the inner workings of the body. They were regarded as the pinnacle of medical practice and were rated the most highly by the population. Finally, apothecaries examined patients and then made and supplied medicines. However, a few doctors undertook more than one of these roles or specialised in a particular area of practice (e.g. mental illness). The term 'general practitioner' was not used until the 1820s.

During the Middle Ages, the word 'nurse' referred to women who were employed to look after children. They were generally classed as servants, although by Shakespeare's time the word had acquired the additional meaning of a woman who cared for the sick. This duality of meaning continued into Victorian times, so ancestors described in a census, for example, as a nurse may not have the role that we would expect today. Similarly, women caring for those who were ill might be referred to as sick attendants or doctors' assistants, rather than nurses. Before 1919, hospital nurses did not necessarily have any professional training or qualifications.

By an Act of Parliament, from 1902 all midwives were registered with the Central Midwives Board on a Midwives Roll. Before then some of them were trained and registered with individual maternity hospitals (known as lying-in hospitals). Until the 1930s, you may find 'handywomen' mentioned in records such as the census: they helped women give birth, but did not have any special training.

Pharmacists were known as chemists and/or druggists, and began filling a need for making and supplying medicines in the eighteenth century after apothecaries became recognised as medical professionals and focused less on their supply role.

Hospitals

In medieval times healthcare was provided by religious houses, some of these erected specialist buildings called infirmaries or hospitals. St Thomas's Hospital in London, for example, was originally run by Augustinian monks and nuns when it was founded in the twelfth century.

Following the dissolution of the monasteries, a series of voluntary hospitals was set up to care for the sick and needy and were run privately by charities and benefactors. Inevitably, certain areas were better provided for than others. Around the eighteenth century, some hospitals in larger cities began to specialise in terms of the patients they would take, for example, seamen, pregnant women ('lying-in' hospitals), orphans, or those with venereal disease. People with mental illness had always tended to be treated separately in lunatic asylums or madhouses (see Chapter 15).

Voluntary hospitals were run by a board who generally decided which patients should be admitted, but as the nineteenth century unfolded, medical staff acquired progressively more authority over the running of these establishments. Away from the voluntary sector, hospitals were also created by local government, and infirmaries arose under the auspices of the Poor Laws, although workhouses often had some quasi-medical functions as well. From about the 1860s some general practitioners oversaw the medical needs of smaller communities via cottage hospitals.

So, by the time that the National Health Service was created in 1950, there were a range of hospital services available with varying historical origins, and some provided free care and some did not. One thing the NHS achieved quickly was the provision of reasonable standards of free hospital access for everyone, with most existing hospitals being brought under public ownership.

St Bartholomew's Hospital in the early years of the nineteenth century. It is the oldest hospital in London and was founded in 1123 as part of a monastery.

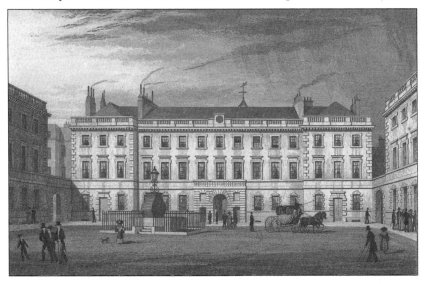

Chapter 2

FINDING A CAUSE OF DEATH

When tracing your ancestors, the further back in time you travel the less likely it becomes that you will find any details about the circumstances of an individual's death. As many family historians discover to their frustration, it is often difficult enough trying to find a date of death, let alone any specific details of the events leading up to it. So whilst you might find a newspaper account, memorial inscription, or correspondence describing the death of an ancestor in the nineteenth century, you would be much more fortunate to find anything similar for the eighteenth century.

Nevertheless, with these limitations in mind, records concerned with a person's death can yield substantial and very interesting information about an ancestor and there are a variety of sources that may assist you. Most of them relate to the deaths of individuals, but some may also describe his or her treatment. It goes without saying that if you have your own family sources, such as letters, diaries or recorded interviews with relatives, they can offer a uniquely detailed and personal insight into an ancestor's demise.

This chapter is a form of checklist for some of the more important sources of information about your ancestors' last hours that you should be aware of. A number of subscription websites offer various indexes to deceased persons including www.ancestry.co.uk , www.findmypast.co.uk, www.thegenealogist.co.uk , and www.familyrelatives.com. The content of these websites changes quite frequently so it is worth looking to see what they offer.

Death Certificates

The compulsory civil registration of births, marriages and deaths commenced in 1837 for England and Wales, 1855 for Scotland, and 1864 for Ireland. Death certificates have changed in format and content over the years, but they have always provided space for a doctor to record cause of death. Sometimes the duration of an ancestor's last illness is recorded as well, e.g. 'diabetes – three months'; a note about a coroner's inquest may also be given. However, the cause given can be very vague (e.g. 'paralysis') or difficult to interpret because medical terminology has changed (e.g. 'exhaustion of the vital powers'). When an elderly person died in the nineteenth century, doctors might simply ascribe death to their advanced years, and not look for a more definitive diagnosis. For example, when 72-year-old Grace Martin died in August 1839, her cause of death was given as 'natural decay'. Other similar phrases used included 'old age', 'elder decline', and 'senility'. The last of these may sometimes imply an element of mental deterioration, but not necessarily. The word 'debility' was often used to describe people who had become weak or infirm especially, but not exclusively, in old age.

Copies of death certificates are available from the General Register Office (GRO) for England and Wales and many of those are indexed by name at the free website www.freebmd.org.uk as well as on the subscription genealogy websites mentioned above; of these, only the Ancestry website includes Irish death indexes. There is also a

According to his memorial at St Thomas's Church, Cricket St Thomas in Somerset, Horatio Hood died in Shanghai, China, in 1881. He has no overseas death certificate, but his obituary in a local newspaper reveals the cause of death – smallpox.

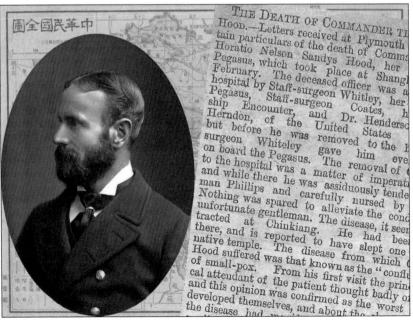

subscription site offering an index to Scottish death certificates at www.scotlandspeople.gov.uk.

Nonetheless, many family historians will have encountered the disappointment of knowing the approximate date of an ancestor's death, but not being able to find a death certificate. Sometimes it is because you cannot clearly identify an individual from a range of possibilities due to a lack of detail, but on other occasions it may be because the death was not registered – especially in the early years of registration. However, there are other reasons. In particular, if there was no corpse then there will be no death certificate, so, for example, ancestors who went down with a ship or were buried under a landslide, and whose bodies were never found, will not have a death certificate. In the past, a British death certificate was also not usually granted if a person died abroad.

Registers of Deaths Abroad and at Sea

The GRO compiled separate registers of British citizens who were born, married or died abroad, including on board ships. There were various mechanisms by which these deaths were notified. The resulting registers are all held at The National Archives (TNA) at Kew, and include:

- RG 32 – Miscellaneous Foreign Returns (1831–1969). Notifications of deaths of British citizens abroad from officials overseas; often not in English.
- RG 33 – Foreign Registers and Returns (1627–1960). Compiled from notifications via British churches, embassies, and politicians abroad.
- RG 35 – Miscellaneous Foreign Death Returns (1791–1921). Includes foreign death certificates and death registers kept by British embassies.
- RG 36 – Registers and Returns of Births, Marriages and Deaths in the Protectorates etc. of Africa and Asia (1895–1965). Civil registration notices related to British citizens.

These four series have been indexed by name and are available online via subscription websites such as www.bmdregisters.co.uk. Once you have found the person in this index, you can order copies of original papers via the GRO, but note that they do not necessarily always include a cause of death.

There is a GRO 'marine' register for deaths at sea on British ships from 1837, with some data coming from the logs of ships. This Marine Register has been indexed and is available on subscription websites such as www.thegenealogist.co.uk where it is listed as 'Overseas Marine Deaths'.

There are a series of separate registers of civilian seamen's and passengers' deaths at sea (see Chapter 3).

Obituaries

Whilst obituaries tend to focus on the date of a person's death and, if you're lucky, their lifetime achievements, they do sometimes mention cause of death. It is important to look in more than one newspaper, as different papers often record different details. For example, the *Gentleman's Magazine* for January 1820 describes the death of Frances Thomasine, Countess Talbot on 20 December the preceding year:

> At the Phoenix Park, Dublin, Frances Thomasine Countess Talbot, in her 38th year. Her ladyship's disorder was an inflammation of the bowels. The rapidity of the progress of this dreadful visitation, left scarcely a pause between alarm and despair. On Tuesday her complaint assumed a character of danger and on Wednesday Her Excellency's state was such as to preclude all hope of recovery.

Obviously, newspapers and general periodicals are a good source for obituaries, but do consider looking at specialised regular publications with a more restricted audience. These may include obituaries, and here are some examples of the types of sources you might look for:

- Deaths of military personnel are usually recorded officially, but less formal publications devoted to a particular armed service may yield helpful extra information. Service magazines, such as the Royal Marines' journal *Globe and Laurel* (from 1892), can be a good source of obituaries.
- Magazines and journals from charities and trades unions often include obituaries for leading members. For instance, the RNLI publication, the *Lifeboat*, was first published in 1852. It records circumstances in which its volunteers died during rescues and the obituaries of significant figures in the service (e.g. former coxswains).
- Churchgoers' deaths may be recorded in local parish magazines. However, many religious denominations had regular national publications that may include members' obituaries, such as the *Monthly Repository* which was a publication of the Unitarian Church (1806–38).
- Publications devoted to a specific trade, profession, or learned society may record detailed obituaries of members. The *Pharmaceutical Journal*, for example, began in 1841 and records obituaries of many British pharmacists.

Coroners' Inquests and Legal Proceedings

The law might be invoked in certain situations where details of a person's health or the circumstances of their death could be made explicit. This includes criminal trials where the charge was murder (or manslaughter) and these cases are discussed in Chapter 12.

Where there was an unexpected death or suspicion of foul play, a coroner's inquest might be called for. Surviving coroners' inquests are often kept in local or county archives, but a great many have not survived. Fortunately, newspapers often report cases where the original record is now missing. TNA holds many inquest records because they were often reported to the Court of King's Bench as well as documented locally; TNA also has certain inquests related to individual institutions. There is a research guide to help you find these inquests: look under 'coroner' at www.nationalarchives.gov.uk/records/atoz. Before the late nineteenth century, inquests were often short and simple. Here is the complete text of an inquest relating to one of my own ancestors from the seventeenth century:

> An inquiry indenture taken at the town and county of Poole, the nineteenth day of May in the fifth year of the reign of King William and Queen Mary over England etc and in the year of our Lord 1693. Before Moses Durell Jr and Joseph Wadham, coroners of the said town and county, upon view of the dead body of Robert Wills, late of the town and county aforesaid, fisherman, lying dead within the said town and county by the oaths of Richmond Smith, Robert Wharton, Richard Brinknam, Oliver Paine, Philemon Pike, Thomas Rowse, Nicholas Rowse, William Malbine, William Rooks, John Scrivener, John Winsor, Zephaniah Thompson and Richard Williams – good and lawful men.
>
> Who say upon their oaths that the said Robert Wills, being alone in his boat between Brownsea and Poole, and being aged and feeble, did by some accident fall into the sea and was drowned, and thus the jury aforesaid by giving their oaths aforesaid do say that the said Robert Wills came by his death and no otherwise, to their knowledge nor dealings. In witness whereof as well the coroners aforesaid as the jurors aforesaid, have hereunto set their hand the day and year above written. [Spelling and punctuation modernised.]

In the event of a major loss of life there may be an official inquiry – after a shipwreck, for example, or an industrial accident or train crash. If a person died intestate, then the administration drawn up to dispose of their worldly goods might mention the cause of their death. Sometimes the legality of a will was disputed on account of the alleged insanity of the will's author or of a beneficiary (see Chapter 15).

Registers of Parish Burials

Before the advent of civil registration of deaths, parish burial registers occasionally yielded information about an individual's fate. This is perhaps most widespread for persons who drowned – and you might see a note to this effect in the margin if the body was recovered for interment. But you can also find occasional notes next to an entry such as 'from the asylum', 'being hanged', 'fever', 'smallpox' and so forth. It depended on the whim or interest of the priest or churchwarden.

It was often the unusual forms of death that attracted the most detailed notes. For example, Elizabeth Burton, aged 5 years from Colton in Norfolk, was 'burnt to death by a dog throwing her into the fire' in 1781. Whereas the parish register at Whitkirk, Yorkshire, records in 1793 that William Coltass was 'slain by a tree falling upon him'.

Very rarely an individual parish documented the causes of death for most of its inhabitants, and you may be fortunate enough to discover an ancestor who lived in one of these areas. The parish of St Cuthbert's, North Meols, Lancashire, for example, listed the cause of death for most of the population in the burials register from May 1789 until 1801 and to read through it is a fascinating study. Here are some consecutive entries from the register for 1792, with my suggestions of a likely modern diagnosis in brackets:

> 5th Jan, Margaret Goore, aged 81 years, weakness [perhaps a stroke].

> 28th Jan, Thomas Abram, aged 2 years, ulcerated throat [probably diphtheria].

> 18th Feb, John Leigh, aged 61 years, jaundice [hepatitis, liver cancer].

> 23rd March, John Halsall, aged 5 years, smallpox.

> 26th March, John Balshaw, aged 36 years, a consumption [tuberculosis].

> 29th March, Thomas Leadbetter, aged 3 years, inward convulsions [epilepsy or a childhood infection].

Many parish burials have been indexed on the genealogy subscription websites noted at the beginning of this chapter, but you can also access many for free via www.familysearch.org and www.onlineparishclerks. org.uk. The subscription website www.bmdregisters.co.uk incorporates Nonconformist burial records. Look also at the memorials section below.

Memorials and Gravestones

Most memorials do not reveal the cause of an individual's death. However, occasionally they do. As with parish registers, it is often the unusual or dramatic causes of death that are recorded. One of the most disturbing, perhaps, is the gravestone of 17-year-old Richard Parker, in Pear Tree Parish Church, Southampton. He died at sea in 1884 'after nineteen days dreadful suffering in an open boat in the Tropics, having been wrecked in the yacht *Mignonette*', but the memorial goes on to explain that 'he was killed and eaten by Tom Dudley and Edwin

William Rogers' memorial in Gosport is the only source that records his cause of death – he died from cholera while in India.

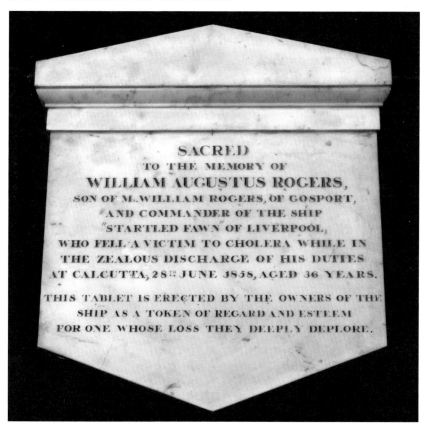

SACRED
TO THE MEMORY OF
WILLIAM AUGUSTUS ROGERS,
SON OF M. WILLIAM ROGERS, OF GOSPORT,
AND COMMANDER OF THE SHIP
"STARTLED FAWN" OF LIVERPOOL,
WHO FELL A VICTIM TO CHOLERA WHILE IN
THE ZEALOUS DISCHARGE OF HIS DUTIES
AT CALCUTTA, 28TH JUNE 1858, AGED 36 YEARS.

THIS TABLET IS ERECTED BY THE OWNERS OF THE
SHIP AS A TOKEN OF REGARD AND ESTEEM
FOR ONE WHOSE LOSS THEY DEEPLY DEPLORE.

Stephens to prevent starvation'. Similarly, a headstone at Malmesbury Abbey in Wiltshire poetically records the dreadful fate of 33-year-old barmaid Hannah Twynnoy:

> In bloom of life,
> She's snatched from hence
> She had no room
> To make defence
> For tyger fierce
> Took life away
> And here she lies in a bed of clay
> Until the Resurrection Day.

Other memorials reveal the sadly more commonplace causes of death such as the tragic memorial to Mary, Cecilia, and Augusta, the three infant daughters of William and Mary Knight of Steventon who 'were cut off by scarlet fever' within a few days of each other in 1848. The gravestone of Elizabeth Barnard at All Saints Church, Hinton Ampner, reports her much-lamented death 'in child bed' in 1807; Barnard Turner is buried at Therfield church and his memorial describes how he 'died by a fall from his horse 15th June 1784 aged 42'.

Some memorials hint at medical details without being explicit – phrases such as 'after a long struggle' or 'following prolonged illness' being quite commonly found. Some texts go a little further. An intriguing memorial at Holy Trinity Church, Gosport, recounts the death in 1779 of William Redfearn of the East India Company who 'returned from India for the benefit of his health, and in vain tried all that was recommended to him in England, Wales and the south of France, but died on the Motherbank on board the *Norfolk*, East Indiaman, just after he had embarked with an intention of returning to India, worn out by long illness in the 29th year of his age'.

The final resting places of many ancestors are recorded on subscription websites such as www.deceasedonline.com and in the National Burial Index which is available at many county archives and libraries or on subscription via www.findmypast.co.uk. Websites devoted to a particular cemetery may have an online index to memorials, and some examples are given in Chapter 27.

Newspapers

As noted above, newspapers are a source of obituaries, but they have value that goes beyond the death notices for individuals. The papers report events that may have involved the death of your ancestor such as court cases and coroners' inquests, or in which he or she was inadvertently caught up. Reporters describe situations where many people died and where individuals might not be mentioned by name such as fires, shipwrecks, civil unrest, or environmental disasters. For example, Samuel Busby's death certificate shows he died on Christmas Eve 1874 at Woodstock in a rail accident. National newspapers such as *The Times* and *Illustrated London News* identify the incident as the Shipton-on-Cherwell train crash. Samuel is not mentioned by name, but the papers describe the circumstances of the crash, and report that thirty-four passengers died. Local newspapers such as the *Banbury Guardian* add more detail. In February the following year, the results of a public inquiry into the incident were also covered by the press.

Whenever you're thinking of consulting newspapers, don't forget to look at both national and local papers. Sometimes you may need to consider foreign newspapers – for example, if an ancestor died abroad or at sea.

Local and regional archives can help with finding locations of newspapers. They have often compiled indexes to their local newspapers, but many digitised versions can be searched via the subscription sites

Crowds gather in the aftermath of the Shipton-on-Cherwell train crash, in which Samuel Busby died, as depicted in a contemporary newspaper.

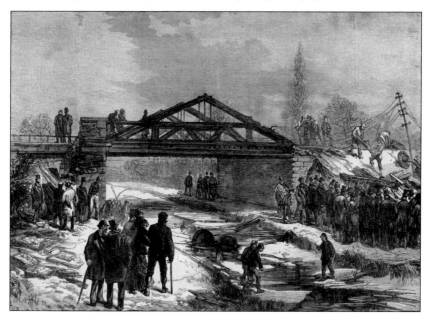

www.britishnewspaperarchive.co.uk and http://newspaperarchive.com. There is also a list of many digital newspaper archives from around the world at: http://en.wikipedia.org/wiki/Wikipedia:List_of_online_ newspaper_archives. Some national newspapers are available online including *The Times* from 1785 onwards at http://gale.cengage.co.uk/ times.aspx/ and libraries frequently have access to this. The Genealogist (www.thegenealogist.co.uk) has a good collection of Victorian editions of the *Illustrated London News*.

Hospitals , Workhouses, and Asylums

Records relating to inpatients treated in British hospitals have survived in piecemeal fashion, and they are dispersed all over the country, although a high proportion of records have been destroyed. The HospRec database, compiled by the Wellcome Trust, indexes the various records known to be available by name or location of hospital, and shows you where they are now located; it can be accessed at www.nationalarchives. gov.uk/hospitalrecords. This database includes records for asylums as well as general hospitals. HospRec incorporates many documents listed in the National Register of Archives (www.nationalarchives.gov.uk/nra) and Access to Archives (www.nationalarchives.gov.uk/a2a), but you should search both of these as well if you don't find what you're looking for because HospRec is not totally comprehensive.

If you are fortunate enough to locate surviving records for the hospital that interests you, you may find patient-specific documents, such as admissions registers but they often provide simply a list of names and admission dates, although some are more detailed. Many hospital records are 'administrative' papers which rarely refer to individual patients, and hence often prove disappointing to the family historian. Having said that, you won't know until you look. Few examples of what we now call case notes survive, i.e. the detailed day-by-day record by doctors of a patient's care.

You should appreciate that even if you do find records for the hospital of interest, the archive holding them is unlikely to allow you access to any patient-specific documents less than a hundred years old (unless you are the patient in question).

Some hospital records have been made available online. The Historic Hospital Admission Registers Project has copied and indexed admissions registers and some case notes from four children's hospitals in London and Glasgow dating from 1852 to 1914. You need to register with the website to see all the information available at www.hharp.org but you can then look for ancestors who may have been admitted in childhood.

For example, 1-year-old Harriet White from Clapham was admitted to Great Ormond Street in 1886 and diagnosed with tuberculosis. She spent two days in hospital, but sadly died there on 25 November. Similarly, admissions and discharges for Salisbury Infirmary 1761 to 1832 are available at www.findmypast.co.uk (subscription needed).

The various records kept by workhouses and Poor Law unions after 1834 may contain details of the health and/or deaths of the people they supported. Illness was a common reason for being admitted, or needing financial support ('relief') in the community. Some of these records will be held by local or county archive services, but TNA holds a collection of formal communications with Poor Law unions in its series MH 12 and selected unions' archives have been indexed online. You can thus use TNA's Discovery service to search for individuals mentioned in the records, http://discovery.nationalarchives.gov.uk. Type in a surname and restrict the search to series MH 12. Look under 'workhouses' in TNA's list of research guides for more information, www.national archives.gov.uk/records/atoz.

Here are two examples from TNA's collection:

Report from Colyton, Devon, in the Axminster Poor Law Union, 1842:

Jacob Birch was a pauper for about 12 months previous to his death last June. He was between 60 and 70, and had a wife some years younger who was considered able-bodied as she went out washing and charring. He received relief on account of rheumatism at first and afterwards with cancer from which he died … During the last seven weeks of his life he received in relief, two shillings in money, two loaves of bread worth 8d a loaf, 2lbs of mutton worth 2s 6d, and a pint of port wine weekly, value 2s 6d.

[TNA ref MH 12/2096/293]

Letter from the Poor Law Board to the Southwell Union, Notts, 1857:

I am directed by the Poor Law Board to state that they have had under their consideration the case submitted to them from the guardians of the Southwell Union on the 17th inst with regard to the funds chargeable with the relief given to William Jackson, now deceased.

It appears that the relief afforded to the pauper was rendered necessary by sickness and does not appear that the sickness (namely typhus fever) was such as would probably have satisfied any justices that it would produce permanent disability … and that consequently the cost of both the relief and the burial are cast upon the Common Fund.

[TNA ref MH 12/9531/254]

The 'records and resources' section of The Workhouse website at www.workhouses.org.uk will assist you in finding local records, as well as explaining the background to Poor Laws and workhouses.

The records kept by lunatic asylums are discussed in Chapter 15.

Military Records

A large number of military records refer to the deaths or injury of individuals and the majority of the originals are now kept at TNA. There are official records kept by surgeons, hospitals, and senior officers, as well as archives relating to the military service of individuals, prisoners of war, gallantry medals and awards, and specific armed forces operations, to cite a few examples. In addition, there may also be unofficial (personal) records written by individuals such as correspondence, journals, and published books. TNA has research guides on its website that give details of its holdings, www.nationalarchives.gov.uk.

The wealth of information on offer makes it difficult sometimes to know what is available, where it is kept, and how best to use it. In Chapter 25, some examples are given but if you have Royal Navy, army, Royal Marines, or Royal Air Force ancestors you should consult the specialist books in this Pen & Sword series that discuss military records in detail.

Employment Records

Where they have survived, some civilian employment-related records may shed light on the deaths of individuals. A good example is the various records related to the merchant navy, which was one of Britain's biggest employers in the nineteenth and early twentieth centuries. These are discussed in a separate book in this series – *Tracing Your Merchant Navy Ancestors* by Simon Wills. Suffice it to say that various government registration schemes and their associated paperwork sometimes recorded the fates of individuals, and that some shipping company records have also survived. However, you may find employment records from all sorts of employers such as mining companies, railways, the civil service, charities, and so on.

Specific Medical Problems

Before the twentieth century, medical journals often identified by name the patients that doctors described in the published cases. Finding ancestors in these journals is not easy because many of them have not been indexed. However, if there was an outbreak of an infectious disease in a particular community, it may be worth looking at medical journals of the appropriate era to see if a local doctor wrote up his experiences. When cholera first broke out in Britain in 1831, a journal called the *Cholera Gazette*, for example, recorded the fates of many named persons as doctors described their attempts to treat them.

Occasionally a specific medical problem attracted the attention of officialdom. For example, local authorities used the Licensing Act of 1902 to compile indexes to habitual drunkards who ought not to be served alcohol (see Chapter 4), and Royal Navy sailors with venereal disease in the era of wooden ships were often identified by name in the ship's paybook if a doctor was called on board to treat them.

Epidemic Statistics

An epidemic is an infection that affects the whole country, as opposed to a local outbreak confined to one community. Knowledge of the years in which particular epidemics occurred may enable you to speculate on the cause of an ancestor's death – particularly if your only source for a date of death is, say, a parish register. Cholera and plague are examples of infections that have invaded Britain in this way and the chapters devoted to these diseases will show you the principal years affected. Many infections do not usually operate as epidemics and continue to affect the population to a similar extent year on year (e.g. venereal disease, chest infections), whilst others may be more common in one year than another in a particular community if conditions are right for a localised outbreak (e.g. typhus, dysentery). Local archives may hold information about historical outbreaks of disease or disasters where many people died within their catchment area.

Chapter 3

ACCIDENTS AND DISASTERS

In the era before civil registration, deaths by accident are more likely to be documented than many other more common means of dying – particularly if many people were killed or the death was a bizarre or unlikely one. These apparently random, cruel tricks of fate touched a chord in the communities affected and people were often keen to record the events for posterity on gravestones and memorials; in newspapers and parish records.

Although accidents are, by definition, caused by misfortune, a number of factors can increase the threat. Perhaps the most obvious risk factor is the nature of an ancestor's employment, since some jobs carry inherent dangers. Coalminers, for example, are exposed to the risk of explosions, gassing, and being buried alive. The Coal Mining History Resource Centre has a valuable database of these tragic events since 1600 with an index of those who have died in mining related incidents, www.cmhrc.co.uk. Many children worked down the mines as well as adults, as can be seen from this report in the *Atheneum*, 1823:

> On Monday night last (Oct. 20), Whitehaven was thrown into the utmost agitation by an awful explosion of fire-damp from the William Pitt coal-mine, belonging to the Earl of Lonsdale. No less than 15 men, 16 boys, and 2 girls have come to a premature death by this catastrophe. It is generally supposed that one of the workmen occasioned the explosion by carelessly removing the cylinder of his lamp. There were also 17 horses killed, but some of their drivers escaped.

Quarry working was another line of work where employees were particularly susceptible to accidents, as the following account from the *Windsor and Eton Express*, 1827, reveals:

On Wednesday, the 21st ult., the coroner took an inquest on the body of Joseph Causton, at Tottenhoe. It was stated in evidence that the deceased was a maker of whiting, and on the Monday previous went with a horse and cart for some chalk to a pit on Dunstable Downs, where he was found buried between two and three feet under a large quantity of chalk that had fallen on him. It did not appear that any person had been with him, but James Smith, who follows the same occupation as the deceased, went to the same pit, and seeing the deceased's horse and cart there, and his jacket lying on the ground, suspected what had happened, and went for assistance to remove the chalk, under which the deceased was found as above stated. It is thought he must have been under the chalk four or five hours. Verdict accordingly.

However, the risks posed to certain other groups may be less obvious and more rarely fatal, so that you only become aware of them when an ancestor is affected. For example, one of my ancestors, James Wills, was a shipwright who in 1900, according to his gravestone, was 'crushed by the yacht *Lyonesse* which fell on him in Looe Harbour'.

The weather can play an important part in causing accidents: storms wreck ships and destroy houses, and excessive rain causes communities to flood. Occasionally the weather literally strikes down individuals – a memorial plaque at St Mary's Church, Lambeth, explains that William Bacon 'was killed by thunder and lightning at his window, July 13th 1787, aged 34 years'.

Another important influencer of the likelihood of accidents is extremes of human age. Both the very young and the very elderly are less likely to recognise danger and to respond to it appropriately.

From 1837 onwards it is possible to analyse the causes of death given on death certificates for England and Wales and provide some statistics related to accidents. For example, in 1865, there were 490,909 deaths registered, but the total number attributable to accidental causes was 15,533 (3 per cent of the total). Accidents were separated from deaths caused by disease, or by deliberate or criminal action (e.g. suicides, murder). The causes of accidental deaths break down as follows:

Fractures and contusions	6,843
Drowning	2,823*
Burns and scalding	2,713
Suffocation	1,309
Poisoning by accident	273
Gunshot	112
Cut or stab	93
Other accidental modes	1,367

* Figures for drowning include only those cases where a body was retrieved and thus a death certificate was issued; the majority of people drowned at sea were never found so this figure is a considerable underestimate of the real number.

Water, Fire, and Falls

Sometimes everyday living is violently interrupted by unexpected tragedy. Drowning is a good example of a form of accidental death that was a lot more common in the past than it is now. A casual perusal of coroners' inquests from before the mid-nineteenth century often reveals a large number of drownings, even in areas away from the coast. John Choppinge, an infant from Hertford, drowned in the family pond in April 1560 when he followed a gosling into the water. In October 1659, Corporal Robert Greene tried to cross the Mersey on horseback but the animal slipped and 'turned over several times'; the horse survived, but not Greene.

Water was a quick and cheap method of long-distance travel by river, by canal, or by sea for our ancestors. Yet, as the two examples above show, accidents on ships and boats are only part of the story behind drownings. People tripped on riverbanks, bridges, and quays; they slipped whilst washing themselves or their clothes in the river; they fell down wells; they attempted to cross rivers when it wasn't safe; they tried to rescue dogs or livestock caught in deep water.

In 1825, the *Salisbury and Winchester Journal* reported:

> Mrs. Cording, a farmer's wife, of Huish Champflower, Somersetshire, having become a Ranter, was so deluded by the doctrines of that sect as to become deranged; she was consequently sent to an asylum for lunatics, from which she escaped last week, and returned to her mother's at Batheaston. Her husband went to see her, when she immediately rushed out of the house, and threw herself into a fish-pond. The husband plunged in, but was unable to rescue her, and both were drowned.

It is notable that few people could swim until comparatively modern times, even those who spent their lives on the water such as fishermen and sailors. When I was a boy, an old fishermen recounted his ancestors' attitudes, many of whom believed, he said, that swimming would only prolong the inevitable agony of drowning if you ended up in the water.

Note that before the law changed in 1808 many parishes felt that drowning, and particularly drowning at sea, was an unnatural death and so insisted on burial in unconsecrated ground. In this case there would usually be no entry in the parish burial register.

Fire was another significant hazard, especially in the era when most houses were made of wood. The Great Fire of London in 1666 stands out as the most notorious example. Remarkably few people seem to have died in this famous conflagration, although many bodies were probably not retrieved, and many more of the resulting homeless may have died subsequently of exposure, disease, and starvation.

In 1727, there was an infamous fire in the village of Burwell, Cambridgeshire. About 140 people had gathered to see a theatrical performance in a barn and once they were inside, the building's doors were sealed, probably to stop anyone getting in without paying. That year's parish register describes what happened:

> At about 9 o'clock on the evening of September 8th 1727, fire broke out in a barn, in which a great number of persons were met together to see a puppet show. In the barn were a great many loads of new light straw. The barn was thatched with straw which was very dry, and the inner roof was covered with old dry cobwebs, so that the fire like lightning flew around the barn in an instant. There was but one small door, which was close nailed up, and could not easily be broken down. When it was opened, the passage was so narrow and everybody so impatient to escape that the door was presently blocked up, and most of those that did escape, which was but very few, were forced to crawl over the bodies of those that lay in a heap by the door.
>
> Seventy-six perished immediately and two more died of their wounds within two days … The fire was occasioned by the negligence of a servant who set a candle and lanthorne [lantern] in or near a heap of straw which lay in the barn.

Falls and blows are a common cause of death. For example, the parish burial register records that James Clegg from Pilsworth in Lancashire was 'killed by a fall from a Hayloft' in 1806. Falls from horses are one of the more common of this type of accident. The following account is from the *Bath Journal*, April 1773:

> Yesterday as Robert Heddington Esq. of the Broad Walk, Southwark, was riding an unruly horse, the beast suddenly took fright near the Obelisk in St. George's Fields, and ran away with him, whereby he was thrown off, and his head pitching against the rails, his neck was dislocated, and he was otherwise so much bruised that he died instantly.

Transportation

Road, rail and airline crashes are relatively recent phenomena, but shipping disasters have been with us since antiquity. In Victorian times they were very common – the British Empire owned around 40 per cent of the world's shipping by the middle of the nineteenth century and depended upon it to dominate world trade. In this situation, large numbers of shipwrecks were almost inevitable and Victorian newspapers are filled with accounts of them every week.

In the period 1867 to 1871, for example, there were 7,062 shipping 'casualties' where a merchant ship was at least seriously damaged. In these incidents 2,598 ships were lost completely, along with 8,807 lives. And these figures relate solely to the British coast – they say nothing about the loss of British ships and lives at sea elsewhere in the world.

In Chapter 2, the registers of deaths abroad and at sea are highlighted as possible sources of information about an ancestor who died on a ship. There are a whole series of other resources for the crews of merchant ships lost at sea and these are comprehensibly covered in Simon Wills' *Tracing Your Merchant Navy Ancestors* (Pen & Sword, 2012). However, the most useful series for both seamen and passengers from the late nineteenth century onwards are:

- 1874–88 – Registers of Deaths at Sea of British Nationals (series BT 159 at TNA). Passengers and crew who died are listed in separate volumes for England and Wales, Scotland, and Ireland. They record age, occupation and address of the deceased, and can be searched by name online via www.bmdregisters.co.uk (subscription needed).
- 1891–1972 – Registers and Indexes of Births, Marriages and Deaths of Passengers and Seamen at Sea (BT 334 at TNA). Each entry lists the individual's age and rank, birthplace, and address. These have been digitised and indexed by name at www.findmypast.co.uk (subscription needed).

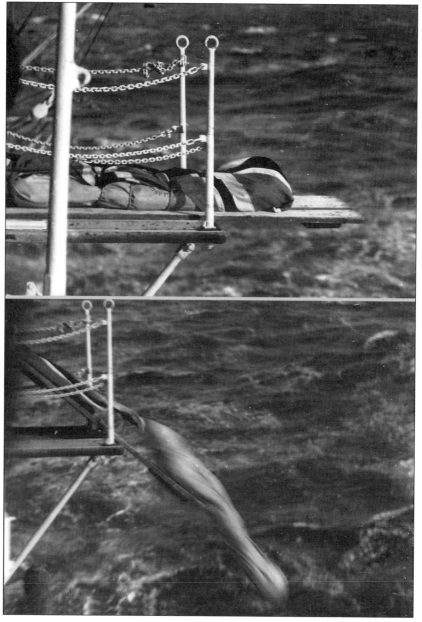

A burial at sea in 1930.

The descendants of seaman William Moffat from Aith in Shetland, for example, have a photograph of him in 1919, but no information on his whereabouts subsequently. Consulting the 1891–1972 records above via www.findmypast.co.uk reveals that he was drowned when the

Newcastle ship SS *Adderstone* sank in the North Sea in 1922. However, note that people could die at sea for all sorts of reasons unrelated to the fate of the ship – through illness, accident, or even murder – and these events should all be recorded in the TNA registers indexes above. Those who died when far from land might be buried at sea.

Memorials dedicated to many people lost at sea can be found by searching the National Maritime Museum's database at http:// memorials.rmg.co.uk.

The other great disaster staple of the Victorian press was the rail crash. The first victim of a railway accident died in 1830. Despite printed warnings to keep clear of the railway lines, William Huskisson, MP for Liverpool, fell under the wheels of George Stephenson's *Rocket*. His leg was so severely mangled that he expired some hours later.

From the 1840s onwards a series of competing railway companies began to establish a network of services across Britain. As the number of railway lines, trains, and passengers escalated, there were inevitably more accidents. Yet, fatal outcomes were much less likely than at sea. In the period 1865 to 1868, for example, there were around a hundred separate accidents involving trains annually and about forty passenger deaths each year as a result. This was not a bad safety rate when the average number of passengers carried on the railways each year was around 270 million.

However, when all railway casualties are counted such as train company employees, deaths due to 'misconduct or want of caution', suicides, people wandering onto the line, and accidents at level crossings the figure is higher. The *Pall Mall Gazette* reported the true figure for 1868:

> The complete official tale of all casualties to life and limb on all the railways of the United Kingdom during the twelve months ending with December last is 212 killed and 600 injured. But among the killed 8 suicides are counted, for which the railways cannot be deemed responsible – unless, indeed, the 8 unfortunates were shareholders.

It is common to find train-crash victims identified in newspaper reports, and the event is likely to be mentioned on a death certificate too. The Railways Archive website at www.railwaysarchive.co.uk catalogues British train crashes by date from 1803 to the present day (look in the Accidents section), and this can be a helpful resource if you know the approximate date or the location.

The first fatal road accident in Britain occurred on 17 August 1896. Arthur Edsall ran over Mrs Bridget Driscoll in south-east London. A

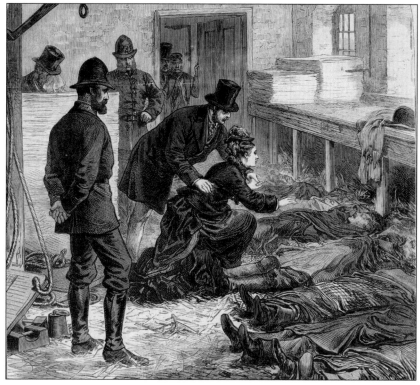

A widow identifying her husband's body after a Victorian rail crash.

petrol vehicle was a great novelty then, and the driver's Roger-Benz car was both very noisy and very slow – it could only manage 4–8mph. Yet somehow the accident still happened. Ironically, the coroner commented that he hoped this unfortunate accident would be the last of its kind.

Plane crashes are almost as old as powered flight. Aviation pioneer Orville Wright killed his third ever passenger, Thomas Selfridge, when his plane nosedived in 1908. This was just five years after his landmark flight with brother Wilbur at Kitty Hawk.

Your Ancestors and Accidents

The survivor of an accident might have to live with some permanent consequences such as disfigurement, amputation, or paralysis and these sad results may sometimes be evident in family photographs. Recovery might be hindered by problems such as wounds, infection or broken bones, but there can also be long-lasting effects such as chronic pain, blindness, or a restricted range of movement. Falls and blows may cause head injuries that lead to epilepsy or mental illness.

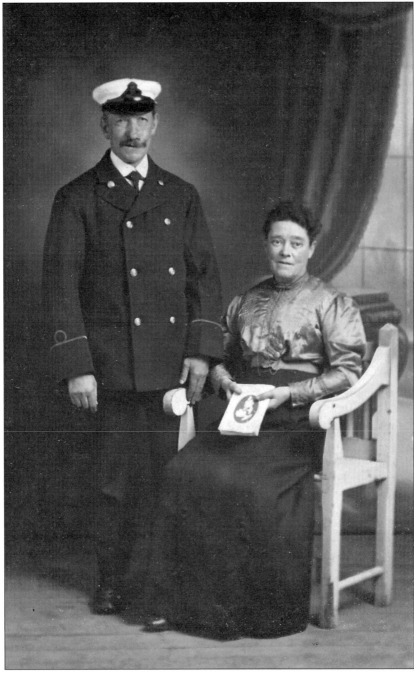

A family photograph of Royal Navy warrant officer John Neal. It shows the facial disfigurement he suffered in a ship's fire in 1899.

Medical problems after the accident could affect a person's future employment, or their ability to care for a family. Until the twentieth century, employers could be quite ruthless and simply dismiss those who were unfit – whether an accident was work-related or not. Yet some employers were sympathetic and offered compensation, support, or even had formal schemes for claiming a pension or relief. For example, Trinity House in London oversaw the employment of ships' pilots and Thomas Boynes of Poole sought compensation from them in 1823. He could no longer work as a pilot 'by reason of a hurt he received in one of his legs as attested by a medical certificate'. The standards of proof required for a successful claim were quite rigorous. Not only did Thomas require a medical certificate, but his MP also had to petition Trinity House personally on his behalf. Nonetheless, Thomas was eventually paid a pension of 10s per month until his death in 1836.

Whatever fate their employers had in store for them, you may find that their surviving records can help you find out more about an ancestor's death – the pit owner's documents in a local archive, for example, or the Royal Navy or merchant ship's logs for sailors.

I mentioned one of my ancestors, James Wills, at the beginning of this chapter, who was crushed by a boat falling on him. That name has been a most unlucky one in my family. Another James Wills, for example, was the victim of an accident in 1842: both of his hands were blown off when a canon exploded on board his ship on a voyage to Quebec. Miraculously, he survived, but perhaps even more miraculously his family rallied around him and he managed to set himself up in business as a very successful shopkeeper and publican. Incredibly, he even went back to sea as a ship's captain in the 1850s. So before the welfare state existed, some victims facing dreadful adversity following an accident could continue to earn a living if they were supported.

If a married man died because of an accident, his wife and children could risk almost immediate homelessness and starvation. In Victorian times the workhouses were made deliberately harsh and uninviting to ensure they were only ever used as a last resort, and so families would try to make their way without seeking workhouse support. However, if there was an accident, other family members might be able to rally round to provide food or shelter, and local people would often hold a collection to help a bereaved family to cope with the immediate aftermath. Details of these collections are often described in local newspapers.

As already noted, there was no burial, or a death certificate, following certain accidents if the body was not retrieved for internment in Britain (e.g. after some drownings, fires, mining accidents, deaths abroad).

Chapter 4

ALCOHOL AND ALCOHOLISM

Alcohol is formed when yeast acts on plant sugars. This process is called fermentation, and often occurs naturally when fruit rots, because yeasts are widespread in the environment. Many early human cultures realised that fermentation could be used to create alcoholic drinks, and it is not surprising that the practice is probably at least 12,000 years old.

Early beverages would have had a low alcohol content because the sugar content of wild fruits and cereals is comparatively low compared to today's varieties which have been selectively bred to make them sweeter. Our ancient ancestors would have produced cloudy looking beers and weak wines that would not have kept well.

British Alcohol Production

The Romans introduced Britons to the forerunner of the pub – the *taberna* – as a roadside place of refreshment. They also established the first grapevines for wine production, although viticulture was already many millennia old by the time of the Roman Empire. Yet this activity has persisted in Britain on a small scale ever since: in 1086, for example, over 600 years after the Romans left, the Domesday Book records 39 vineyards in England.

British beers (or 'ales') were traditionally made from fermented malt, typically produced by allowing barley grain to begin germinating then heating it to stop the growth. A

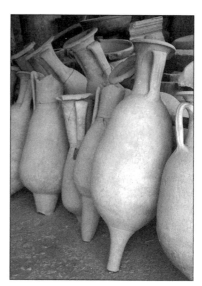

Roman wine storage containers or amphorae.

large number of malthouses grew up to support this industry. Fresh drinking water was not always easily obtainable to our ancestors – especially in urban areas – and so beers were a cheap, more palatable, and safer option. Their low alcohol content meant that family members of all ages could drink beer throughout the day as refreshment, and as freely as we now drink water, tea, or fruit juices. Young children and invalids often drank 'small beer' which had an even lower alcohol content. Beers could also be stored for a few months without going off, so the navy, for example, served beer on board its warships because it kept better than water.

Trouble Brewing

The production of spirits (or 'drams') in Britain did not commence until the introduction of distillation in the seventeenth century. Distillation allowed the creation of whisky in Scotland and Ireland, rum in British colonies in the Caribbean, and gin in England. These potent alcoholic drinks inevitably caused more drunkenness.

Early writers on alcohol, stress the behavioural problems that drunkenness produced for the individual, and these were often seen as offences against God. Jeremy Taylor, Charles I's personal chaplain, wrote a tract, *The Rule and Exercises of Holy Living*, in 1650 that illustrates that not much has changed in over 360 years. He characterised drunkenness by:

1. Apish gestures.
2. Much talking.
3. Immoderate laughing.
4. Dullness of sense.
5. Scurrility, that is wanton jeering or abusive language.
6. A useless understanding.
7. Stupid sleep.
8. Epilepsies, or fallings and reelings, and beastly vomiting.

Although alehouses had been regulated since 1552, anyone could make or sell spirits and they became widely available and were extremely cheap – much cheaper than beer. By the beginning of the eighteenth century there was increasing concern about persistent public drunkenness, and more particularly the resultant widespread lawlessness, violence, and debauchery, especially in the capital. The streets were unsafe, families were neglected, and employers could not get men to do work. Daniel Defoe wrote that even gentlemen found drunkenness fashionable. In some parts of London in the 1720s, an official report noted that as many as one in five houses was a gin shop. Many vendors used a then-famous slogan: 'Get drunk for a penny, and dead drunk for twopence'. In the 1690s, English people had consumed about 800,000 gallons of spirits per year, whereas by 1736 consumption had leapt to an amazing 6 million gallons with no significant increase in the population.

The Gin Act

The Gin Act of 1736 was a poorly designed attempt to reduce the excess consumption of spirits by making it unaffordable to the poor, who were its chief consumers. A duty of 20s per gallon was imposed, together with an annual fee of £50 for all those who sold it. These measures were far too harsh and so were widely ignored: gin and other spirits were still sold but under other names such as 'Knock Me Down' or 'Make Shift'. To evade the need to register premises, many sellers took to roaming the streets, selling gin from barrows or carts. Those who informed on people evading the law risked their lives, as did some of the magistrates who convicted offenders. There were gin riots in cities, and smuggling of spirits from abroad was rife, especially Dutch gin or 'Geneva'.

Some sellers disguised their spirits as medicines by adding a dye and labelling them with instructions such as: 'Take two or three spoonsful of

Many of Hogarth's pictures capture the alcohol excess of eighteenth-century society – this one illustrates the various stages of inebriation.

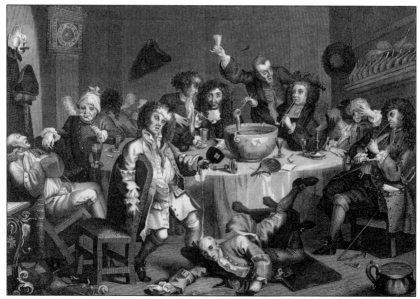

this four or five times a day or as often as the fit takes you.' Apothecaries were allowed to sell spirits for the relief of illness, many of which were traditionally used to treat stomach complaints, and one newspaper records that 'Several apothecaries' shops had so great a call for gripe and cholic waters etc, by the poor sort of people, that the masters were obliged to employ an additional number of hands in serving them.'

It soon became clear that the sheer numbers of offenders meant that the new law was unenforceable. So, in 1743, the Act was repealed after a 'vexatious and unprofitable trial' and replaced with more liberal licensing controls. However, within a few years heavy drinking began to lessen largely for economic reasons. In the 1750s, gin became more expensive because grain prices rose, and at the same time there was a slump in wages. The government also restricted spirits sales to 'respectable' premises and increased the cost of its licences. In 1757, the domestic production of spirits from cereals was made illegal.

Towards the end of the eighteenth century, writers such as William Paley could look back and appreciate that the ill effects of persistent drunkenness extended to a wider sphere than just the drinker. The following quotation is taken from Paley's *The Principles of Moral and Political Philosophy*, 1785:

> By drunkenness is here meant habitual intemperance, although the guilt and danger is applicable in a certain degree to each specific act of intoxication because habit is only a repetition of single instances.
>
> The guilt of drunkenness is to be estimated from the tendency of its mischievous effects:
>
> 1. It leads to acts or words of anger or lewdness; 2. It interferes with the performance of the duties of a man's station; 3. It leads to extravagance; 4. It produces unhappiness to the drunkard's family; 5. It shortens life, and lastly it corrupts by example.

Victorian Temperance

Despite the far less dramatic drinking habits of the population during the nineteenth century, this era saw the birth of the temperance movement. The organisations that formed this were closely linked to Protestant religions and to the Victorian concept of morality, because alcohol loosened the inhibitions and encouraged immoral behaviour. Temperance groups generally aimed to convert drunkards away from drinking, encourage abstinence in the population, and drastically to restrict alcohol sales. In 1837 the New British and Foreign Temperance

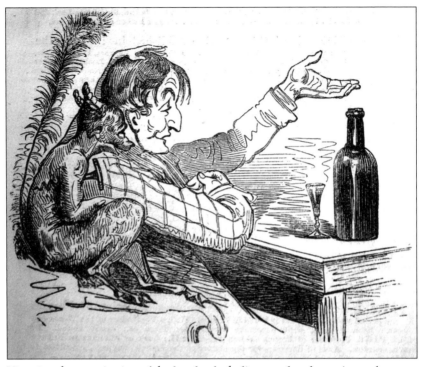

Victorian characterisation of the lonely alcoholic, egged on by an inner demon.

Society reported more than 100,000 members including over 2,000 'cured' drunkards.

An influential publication by James Samuelson, *The History of Drink*, published in 1878 reveals much of the Victorian attitude to alcohol and is also one of the first occasions that the nation's unfortunate global reputation for heavy drinking is mentioned. Samuelson protested that 'no English gentleman now gets drunk', but that despite great improvements amongst the middle classes, there was still far too much drinking, yet little drunkenness except amongst 'fast young men'. The main problem he revealed was the lower classes, especially 'the vicious classes in the great seaports'. These seamen 'whose chief employment is drinking' were the class of society responsible for the country's 'unenviable reputation for drunkenness amongst the nations of the world'.

These pressures from temperance groups and the perception that British people drank too much led to the first legislation to restrict pub opening hours in 1872.

Twentieth-century Regulation

There was further legislation affecting pub opening hours in the twentieth century, particularly in the First World War when the government became concerned that drunkenness was endangering the efficiency of munitions factory workers and other aspects of the war effort. These were later modified again, and until the early twenty-first century pub hours in England and Wales were mainly regulated by legislation from the 1960s.

However, the twentieth century marks the period when the true ill effects of excessive drinking began to be realised, and the advent of health promotion campaigns to promote sensible drinking, and to avoid alcohol when driving. This century also witnessed the discovery that regular intake of small amounts of wine can have health benefits.

Given the disastrous consequences of freely available, cheap alcohol in the eighteenth century, it is interesting that despite initial concerns, the relaxation of pub opening hours in the twenty-first century has thankfully not resulted in population-wide drunkenness on the scale of three centuries ago.

Your Ancestors and Alcohol

Legal proceedings, hospital records, military service documents, and newspaper stories may reveal that an ancestor was overly fond of alcohol. Legal cases may refer to keeping a disorderly house or operating from unlicensed premises. Records of service in the army or navy frequently mention drunkenness as a cause of punishment. In the eighteenth-century navy the standard penalty was twelve lashes, and these offences are often cited in ships' logs for named individuals.

A particular set of records that are preserved in many local archives are photographs and detailed descriptions of habitual drunkards, dating from around 1900. These portray men and women who broke the law whilst drunk, or who were repeatedly arrested for being drunk in public. The photographs were circulated locally and landlords were forbidden to serve them alcohol. There are a set of examples online from the Birmingham Pub Blacklist of 1903–6 on www.ancestry.co.uk (subscription needed).

Alcoholism is rarely given as a specific cause of death on death certificates, but it may be mentioned as a contributing cause. The term 'alcoholism' was not widely used until the late Victorian era. Before then it was referred to by terms such as habitual drunkenness, dipsomania, or persistent intemperance. Alcoholics are likely to die of things such as accidents, strokes, liver disease (e.g. cirrhosis, jaundice), stomach ulcers, fitting, and some forms of abdominal cancer. The NHS Choices website gives a more complete list of medical problems, www.nhs.uk.

Alcohol Throughout History

Society's changeable attitude to alcohol down the centuries is revealed by quotations from writers, politicians, doctors, and personalities.

- 'Who could have foretold from the structure of the brain, that wine could derange its functions?' – Hippocrates, Greek physician (460–377 BCE).
- 'Caesar was the only sober man who ever tried to wreck the Constitution.' – Cato the younger, Roman statesman (95–46 BCE).
- 'The first draught serveth for health, the second for pleasure, the third for shame, the fourth for madness.' – Sir Walter Raleigh, British statesman (1552–1618).
- 'When a man has, by gin drinking, rendered himself unfit for labour or business, he can purchase nothing else; and then the best thing he can do is drink on until he dies.' – Lord Chesterfield, British statesman (1694–1773).
- 'Drunkenness, whoring and swearing: all of them very ill-becoming a gentleman, however custom may have made them modish.' – Daniel Defoe, British writer (1660–1731).
- 'There are some sluggish men who are improved by drinking; as there are fruits that are not good until they are rotten.' – Samuel Johnson, British writer (1709–84).
- 'Wine is the most hygienic and healthful of beverages.' – Louis Pasteur, French scientist (1822–95).
- 'An alcoholic is someone you don't like who drinks as much as you do.' – Dylan Thomas, British poet (1914–53).
- 'One reason I don't drink is that I want to know when I am having a good time.' – Nancy Astor, British politician (1879–1964).
- 'In 1969 I gave up women and alcohol – it was the worst 20 minutes of my life.' – George Best, British footballer (1946–2005).
- 'There are better things in life than alcohol, but alcohol makes up for not having them.' – Terry Pratchett, British author (1948–).

Chapter 5

CANCER

Cancer has become a more visible disease over the past 100 years because people are living longer. We are no longer likely to die from the great killers of the past such as smallpox or TB, and since we are not dying young from the causes that killed our ancestors, we're more likely to develop cancer.

However, cancer is not 'new' – it has always existed and is found, for example, in some Egyptian mummies. The disease's name comes from the ancient Greek physician, Hippocrates, who compared the appearance of a tumour spreading in the body to a crab; the Latin word for crab is 'cancer'.

The Surgeon's Knife

Until a little over 100 years ago, surgery was the only treatment for a cancer tumour that had any chance of success. It makes sense to cut the lump out if you can. Unfortunately, surgery before the twentieth century was crude: the operating environment was not sterile, there were no antibiotics or blood transfusions, and surgical instruments and anaesthetics were primitive. As a result, surgery was painful and disfiguring, and commonly hastened the death of the patient. Those who survived often took a long time to recover.

Apart from poor surgical techniques, operations were often performed far too late in the disease because early diagnosis was not possible. By this time, tumours had already spread too much and surgery was a last resort. This also meant that the disease commonly returned even after the operation, leading many doctors and patients alike to view cancer as incurable.

Yet at least surgery offered some hope. However, for many families – even assuming they could pay for a doctor's visit in the first place – a surgeon was another expense that they simply could not afford.

Quack Treatments

If surgery offered a slim hope, the other treatments for cancer until the end of the nineteenth century offered no hope at all, although they were widely used. They included preparations that burned the tumour or the skin above it. These 'caustics' included hydrochloric acid and caustic soda, and must have caused the poor patients excruciating pain. Many doctors believed that persistent diarrhoea ('purging') was beneficial and used plant remedies to this end and the all-pervasive bloodletting was widely practised well into the nineteenth century for many diseases including cancer.

A whole host of other treatments were applied to the skin or taken by mouth including arsenic, gold, cyanide, iodine, and poisonous plants such as hemlock and belladonna. Mercury, which was used to treat virtually every serious ailment in the eighteenth and nineteenth centuries, was also used. Some doctors advocated bizarre diets such as figs boiled in milk, or eating very large quantities of boiled carrots.

When we look at many of these treatments now, it is alarming how much quackery there was. Unscrupulous doctors took advantage of desperate patients, peddling ineffective cures for which they could charge a great deal. Yet, as one nineteenth-century doctor remarked, 'If I don't prescribe them, the person next consulted will'.

About the only sensible medicine that pre-twentieth century doctors prescribed was opium to treat the patient's pain, something that is still done today, although nowadays the principal active constituent of opium is used instead – morphine.

New Treatments

In the late nineteenth century, X-rays were discovered by William Röntgen in Germany. These mysterious 'beams' were miraculously found to cure some cancers near the surface of the skin without the need for surgery. As X-ray machines became more powerful they were used for more deep-seated tumours as well. The initial enthusiasm was soon marred when researchers realised that X-rays themselves could cause cancer, as well as cure it, if people were exposed to too much. During the twentieth century, this treatment evolved into what we now call radiotherapy. Different forms of radiation were tried, and the treatment was made more focused to avoid healthy parts of the patient's body being exposed to it.

The use of medicines to kill cancer cells is called chemotherapy and, intriguingly, it has its origins in chemical warfare. In the Second World War, doctors studying the effects of mustard gas on army personnel found

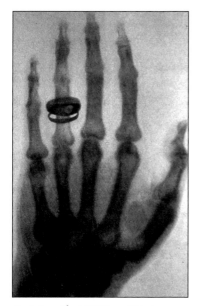

A picture that William Röntgen took of his wife's hand using X-rays in 1896.

changes suggesting it might help to treat lymphoma and leukaemia. A drug named mustine was introduced in the 1940s and proved beneficial to some cancer sufferers. Although the original mustine is now rarely prescribed, many drugs derived from it are still in use.

Early chemotherapy often produced horrendous side effects, which were sometimes lethal. In more recent times, drugs and the ways of giving them have become more selective, and there are antidotes to some of the more serious side effects. This has made them safer, although patients must still be monitored carefully. An important development was the discovery that some common cancers are stimulated to grow by the body's sex hormones, and drugs that block this effect began to be developed in the 1960s.

The development of specialist treatments allowed doctors to specialise too. Cancer began to be treated by oncologists – specialist doctors who understood the disease.

Public Health

In the early twentieth century doctors started writing about the distress that a diagnosis of cancer produced. Cancer took over from TB as the disease that people most dreaded. A lot of the fear was caused by the finality of the diagnosis – the only real option was surgery, which was usually ineffective. Aware of this fear, in an age when doctors and their patients accepted a more paternalistic role for the medical profession, doctors debated the wisdom of revealing the diagnosis at all. If there was nothing that could be done, then maybe it was better for the patient to live a short time in ignorance than to worry that they were bound to die.

This attitude reveals a lot about society's changed approach to health matters in the last hundred years. These days we are educated to recognise that early diagnosis of cancer gives the best hope of a cure, and are taught that if we get sinister symptoms, such as bleeding from the bowel, we should seek medical advice quickly. We know that certain behaviours such as sunbathing and smoking increase the risk of cancer, there are screening programmes for some cancers to detect them early (e.g. breast cancer), and even a childhood vaccine that now reduces the risk of one cancer (cervical cancer).

Yet screening, prevention, and public education are all modern concepts. Today we have fast, free and easy access to information about our health, but until relatively recently doctors were the sole source of medical knowledge in their community. And before the advent of the National Health Service access to this knowledge was not free and universal – it had to be paid for.

In many ways, the story of cancer illustrates how healthcare as a whole has changed for the better in Britain, even though some cancers are still not curable. Patients are more knowledgeable about health issues so can now take more responsibility for themselves including helping to detect cancer early and preventing it. Doctors understand more about the causes of disease so treatments are more carefully targeted, and we expect a partnership and up-to-date information from our doctors when we seek their advice. Even though a diagnosis of cancer may still be frightening, we have a lot more hope of successful treatment than our ancestors ever did.

Your Ancestors and Cancer

The prevalence of cancer in my own family illustrates how the management of the disease has changed over four generations. You may be able to compare medical treatments between eras in your own family by interviewing relatives.

1920s – Surgery the Only Option

My great-grandfather, Richard Wills, was diagnosed with colon cancer in 1921. There was no NHS then, so his working class family scraped together enough money for him to see a surgeon. The surgeon said he would 'open him up' to see what was happening and cut out what he could. In 1922, the surgeon removed a large piece of his bowel and he explained that if Richard survived five days he would be cured of cancer. However, he died three days later.

1950s and 60s – Early Chemotherapy

My brother, Peter, developed childhood leukaemia. Nowadays it is often treated successfully with intensive chemotherapy, but these drugs were in their infancy during Peter's lifetime. He had repeated admissions to hospital and was given high-dose steroids and primitive chemotherapy, which caused many side effects including obesity and multiple infections. He died in 1963.

1970s – Radiotherapy with Surgery

My grandfather, Stephen, had been a lifelong smoker when he was diagnosed with lung cancer in 1974. He had a lung removed surgically – and then radiotherapy to the whole chest to try and remove any remaining cancer. The treatments made him very tired and though they prolonged his life, he died of the cancer in 1976.

1980s – Better Targeted Treatments

My mum, Pat, developed breast cancer and had the tumour surgically removed, she had radiotherapy but carefully targeted to the expected site of the disease which reduced the side effects. She also received hormone chemotherapy to prevent cancer recurrence. These treatments were very successful and completely eradicated the disease.

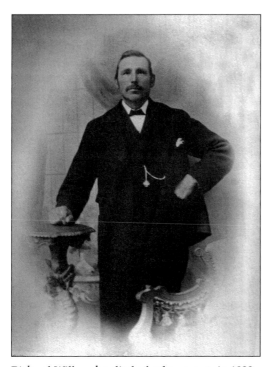

Richard Wills, who died of colon cancer in 1922.

If your research reveals a family history of one kind of cancer that keeps occurring, this awareness may help you to take steps to reduce the risk to those still living.

The commonest term for this disease on death certificates is 'cancer', but you may see other words:

- Carcinoma – the Greek word for crab. Some particular cancers may have long descriptive names, e.g. *carcinoma ventriculi* is stomach cancer.
- Malignant growth – the word malignant means 'spiteful' in Latin and indicates an uncontrolled, serious disease. Conversely a benign growth is not harmful.
- Metastases – cancer that has spread to other parts of the body: a 'metastatic cancer' is not confined to one place.
- Scirrhus, stony, and encephaloid (or medullary) – three basic types of tumour recognised in the nineteenth century.
- Tumour – from the Latin for 'swelling', in former times a tumour usually meant there was a lump that could be seen or felt.

Jaundice

This condition is a symptom of a serious disease of the liver. When the liver is significantly damaged it may no longer be able to excrete bile properly, and so it builds up in the bloodstream making the person's skin turn yellow in colour. The eyeballs are often affected too. Jaundice is a very old medical term which you may find on death certificates, although before 1800 it had many variant spellings including ganders and jaundies. It is also sometimes called icterus. It can be a symptom of a cancer that starts in the liver, but many other cancers spread to the liver and may then cause jaundice (e.g. cancers of the pancreas, bowel, lungs, prostate, breast).

However, there are other causes of jaundice including alcoholism (see Chapter 4), gallstones, yellow fever (Chapter 21), and infections of the liver such as hepatitis A, and Weil's disease (leptospirosis). The liver infections tend to be associated with poor sanitation.

Chapter 6

CHEST CONDITIONS

Medical conditions that affect the lungs are often referred to as chest diseases. The most important of them, historically, has been tuberculosis – which was common and killed a great many – and it is the subject of Chapter 22. However, many other chest conditions have been significant causes of our ancestors' suffering, yet in times gone by doctors may have lacked the skills or knowledge to differentiate between them reliably. For example, it is clear from some contemporary accounts that chest infections, bronchitis, and asthma could be confused. Similarly the word 'tissick' was sometimes used to describe the coughing or wheezing characteristic of many chest diseases, but was also a specific term for tuberculosis. This may mean that a certain amount of latitude has to be granted when interpreting chest diseases on Victorian death certificates.

Asthma

This is a condition where the airways go into spasm, producing attacks of wheeze, cough, and breathlessness. However, in the past the term 'asthma' might be used to describe a whole variety of other breathing complaints.

In 1868, Henry Salter, a London physician, asked one of his patients to describe the causes of her asthma in his book *On Asthma: Its Pathology and Treatment*. Some elements of this description may be familiar to modern sufferers:

> If I walk in the garden when the air is damp and chilly, in ten minutes my breathing becomes sensibly affected. At night if my dress is not securely closed in front, or the bed-clothes well adjusted about my neck and shoulders, a certain degree of asthma presently ensues. It has sometimes happened that I have fallen asleep without having made these necessary arrangements, and the consequence has been that I have awoke

with a fit of suffocation, which, after the removal of the cause, has subsided in the ordinary way. The asthma consequent on cold on the chest (bronchitis) is of a most painful and distressing kind: unlike that produced by cold directly, it often lasts for days. In my childhood I suffered grievously from it; I can remember when I was very little, spending hours at a time on a footstool with my head on a chair as the best means of obtaining rest, together with ability to breathe. Another of the primary causes of asthma with me is change of air.

... The remaining exciting causes – a recumbent posture, laughing, coughing, sneezing, bodily exercise – I call secondary causes ... So great is the tendency of laughing to induce asthma that I have always been obliged, especially in childhood, to avoid it as much as possible on account of its distressing consequences. Coughing, though a symptom of the complaint is also a source of aggravation, and when there is no appearance of asthma is sufficient to call it into existence. A violent fit of sneezing in the summer will produce asthma, otherwise not. I have always suffered from the effects of bodily exercise, especially in childhood; but even at my present age I cannot run a considerable distance, or jump a child, or skip with a skipping-rope, without the occurrence of some asthma.

In Victorian times, asthma attacks could be treated with a wide variety of 'medications' including ipecacuanha (a herb that made people vomit), strong coffee, chloroform, opium, cannabis, and a plant called lobelia, also known as 'asthma weed' or 'Indian tobacco'. Somewhat counter-intuitively, even tobacco was used – the aforementioned Dr Salter remarking that several puffs of a pipe often made patients collapse, but that their wheezy symptoms were usually relieved upon revival! One of his patients corroborates this effect: 'distressing as are the sensations of collapse from tobacco poisoning, they are an unspeakable relief when contrasted with the impending suffocation of asthma'. Similar relief was claimed from burning a piece of paper soaked in saltpetre (or nitre) and asking the patient to inhale its acrid fumes.

To reduce the frequency of attacks, asthma sufferers were encouraged to regulate their diet, move to inland areas to find air that did not provoke their condition, and to take potassium iodide. Other, more bizarre recommendations included frequent cold baths, inhaling the fumes of strong acids every day, and receiving regular electric shocks (Galvanism). Some doctors even believed that asthma was a psychosomatic illness – a form of mental illness with physical symptoms – and focused more on psychiatric treatments.

In the early twentieth century, researchers began to realise that some medicines could be used to open up the airways when they went into spasm. One of the first agents used for this in the western world was the belladonna plant (deadly nightshade), and adrenaline was later used as well. But these medicines were very imprecise in their action so they had lots of side effects; they were also difficult to administer to patients. Eventually in the 1950s and 60s, inhalers were developed to enable more carefully targeted administration of medication to the airways, along with more specific-acting drugs that were better tolerated.

Tobacco Smoking

Tobacco is the dried leaves of the plant *Nicotiana tabacum* which is native to the Americas. It was brought back to Europe in the sixteenth century and soon gained widespread popularity. Sir Walter Raleigh was a famous advocate of smoking. Yet his employer, King James I, considered the practice disgusting – a somewhat ironic judgement from a monarch who never washed his hands and habitually fingered his codpiece in public. Nonetheless, the King pulled no punches and in 1604 he published a *Counterblaste to Tobacco*, in which he declared that smoking was: 'A custome lothsome to the eye, hatefull to the nose, harmefull to the braine, daungerous to the lungs, and in the blacke stinking fume thereof nearest resembling the horrible Stigian smoke of the pit that is bottomelesse.' The King's opinion pre-empted scientific proof of tobacco's most dangerous effects on the lungs by 350 years.

Tobacco was initially smoked in clay pipes, although some people chewed it as a 'quid' which was retained in the mouth for long periods before eventually being spat out. Cigars came into widespread

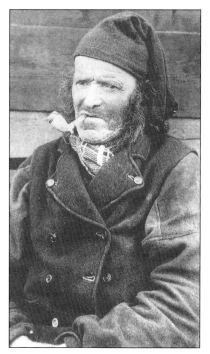

Before cigarettes became widely available, our ancestors used clay pipes to smoke tobacco, as seen in this late Victorian photograph.

use in the early nineteenth century, and cigarettes were first mass-produced towards the end of that century. There was an inexorable rise in smoking, with doctors extolling its health benefits for treating conditions such as tetanus, ear infections, various types of pain, and asthma (as described above). Some physicians even advocated injecting tobacco smoke into the rectum to treat constipation.

However, even in the nineteenth century, medical men began to recognise that tobacco could have harmful effects. Unfortunately, some good work exploring its dangers was drowned out by a tide of ill-founded medical opinions suggesting that smoking caused everything from tuberculosis to insanity. Nineteenth-century arguments about the dangers of tobacco were not helped by, first, a lack of methodical examination of the facts, and, secondly, the great Victorian temptation to moralise about anything deemed pleasurable to the senses.

Tobacco was cheap, easily available, and became socially acceptable across all tiers of society. An ancestor who didn't smoke would have been in the minority. Figures for 1948, for example, show that over half of the British adult population smoked (52 per cent), and two-thirds of all men smoked.

Yet gradually the tide began to turn as the detrimental effects of tobacco were realised. Most notably, studies led by Richard Doll in the 1950s established that smoking was causing the prevailing 'epidemic' of lung cancer. However, the results surprised him – he later revealed that of all the potential causative factors for lung cancer they had looked at, he'd thought tarring of roads would prove to be responsible. From this point onwards a steady flow of research helped establish tobacco's other hazards. We now know that tobacco smoking causes a whole range of diseases. Many of these affect the airways such as lung and throat cancer, bronchitis, and pneumonia, but there are many others such as heart disease, strokes, peptic ulcers, and blindness.

Royal Navy Ancestors

From around 1700 until the twentieth century, the Royal Navy supplied its own men with tobacco. Sailors could take an agreed measure of tobacco and its cost would be set against their future wages. At TNA, you can find tobacco usage carefully recorded in the naval musters and paybooks against the names of individuals who took advantage of this service. It's a curiously specific fact to know about an ancestor from three centuries ago, when you may not know much else about him. It also beggars belief that smoking was allowed on board wooden ships, with their tar-soaked rigging and arsenals of gunpowder – yet fires caused by men smoking tobacco in the navy were virtually unheard of, although some sailors did chew tobacco rather than smoke it. Nonetheless, popular images of sailors in the eighteenth and nineteenth centuries often include a pipe.

Occupational Chest Disorders

Men and women who work for long periods in confined spaces where lots of particles are inhaled can develop lung diseases. The constant breathing in of dust or fibres leads to them becoming lodged deep in the lungs, which react by becoming inflamed and scarred. This damage makes sufferers keep coughing, and the lungs become less efficient so that victims are short of breath. Those affected often die from a chest infection or lung cancer. In former times, some of these diseases had occupational labels for ease of reference, such as miner's lung disease, but contemporary doctors might simply refer to any resulting chest condition as 'bronchitis', or even 'asthma'.

People who worked in mines, cotton and flax mills, flour mills, and malthouses were particularly susceptible, as were grinders, stonemasons, and those who processed metal ores such as foundry workers. In some of these trades the dust was swallowed as well as inhaled, producing indigestion, diarrhoea, or similar symptoms. There are many examples, and it is sadly common to find more than one generation of ancestors following the same trade and dying young. Three specific examples that may be encountered are described below:

- A link between coal mining and lung diseases has been known since at least the sixteenth century. The condition called coal miner's lung is caused by coal dust, and was also called miner's lung disease, spurious melanosis, black phthisis, black lung disease, or anthrocosis.
- Byssinosis was contracted by those who processed plant materials used to make textiles such as hemp, flax, and cotton. Small plant fibres hung in the air and were inhaled in large numbers by the average worker.
- Knife-grinder's disease was also known as grinder's rot or grinder's asthma, and was associated with the cutlery industry in Sheffield. In 1835 it was noted that amongst 2,500 such workers 'the majority die before their 36th year'.

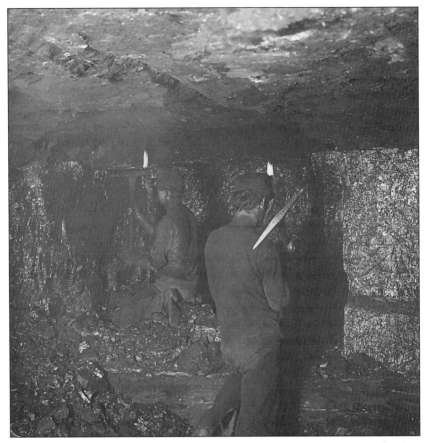

Coal miners were trapped in a confined space and constantly exposed to the dust from the coalface.

Despite the fact that many of their workers died prematurely, employers often resisted any suggestion that their working conditions were responsible.

Anthrax

Anthrax was another disease linked to occupations and was formerly called wool-sorter's disease, charbon, or splenic fever. It is an infection of cattle, sheep, and goats that does not normally spread to humans. However, workers in agriculture, the wool industry, tanning, and butchery were susceptible to it because they handled animal remains extensively. There are three forms of the disease, depending on how it is contracted: via contamination of an open wound on the skin, by swallowing infected material, or by inhaling it.

Inhalation produced the lung form of anthrax which is almost invariably fatal, although people also died from the skin variety of the disease because it often led to blood poisoning (septicaemia). Inhalation can happen after the spores of the causative bacterium, *Bacillus anthracis*, are thrown into the air from shaking animal hides and fleeces, or from grinding animal bones to make fertiliser. The unfortunate victims of an anthrax chest infection soon begin to cough up blood – potentially infecting others in the process – before rapidly expiring. During the Industrial Revolution there were a number of localised anthrax outbreaks in Britain because the processing of animal parts and carcasses became more intensified.

Other Lung Conditions

Five of the most important that you may find on death certificates are:

Bronchitis

This term as we understand it today refers to a condition where the large airways (bronchi) are damaged and become inflamed. This may be short-term due to a viral infection (acute bronchitis), or a long-term reaction to harm from inhaling air contaminated with pollution or tobacco smoke (chronic bronchitis). People with chronic bronchitis have a persistent cough that makes them bring up mucus from the lungs. However, in the past the term 'bronchitis' was frequently used more imprecisely to mean what we would today call a chest infection.

Chest Infections

Chest infections such as pneumonia affect adults or children and are most commonly caused by bacteria. They hastened the demise of many an ancestor, who often succumbed to them as a consequence of other serious or long-term illnesses that left their immune system vulnerable or their lungs weak.

Emphysema

This is a condition where the delicate structure of the lungs is destroyed, particularly the minuscule small air sacs ('alveoli') that enable oxygen to get into the bloodstream. This leaves sufferers short of breath all the time. It's usually associated with long-term inhalation of polluted air, as happens in tobacco smokers or those with industrial illnesses such as coal miner's lung (above).

Pleurisy or Pleuritis

The lungs are surrounded by membranes (pleura) that can become inflamed – often due to infection. This makes it painful to draw breath, cough, sneeze and so forth. Pleurisy is often a sign of an existing chest disease such as tuberculosis, pneumonia, or a physical injury, but it can occur as a complication of other diseases or even by itself.

Whooping Cough

This killed many children in the pre-vaccination era (see Chapter 7).

Chapter 7

CHILDREN, BABIES, AND INFECTION

One of the greatest joys for any couple is the birth of a child, yet parents quickly learn that their children are prone to all sorts of bugs, even at the youngest ages. These days medical attention is easy to access in Britain, but in the past thousands of babies and children died or became seriously ill because of infection every year. These infections varied a lot in their severity, and were more likely in children who were malnourished, but the biggest individual killer was probably smallpox (see Chapter 20). Fortunately, we now immunise children against many of the most serious diseases and, thanks to vaccination, smallpox has been completely eradicated.

Many infections that our ancestors' children suffered from were those such as diphtheria, measles, meningitis, scarlet fever, smallpox, and whooping cough. So there was an increased risk of transmission in places where many children were collected together such as the cramped housing conditions where many families were forced to live side by side, and in schools, orphanages, and workhouses.

Describing Children

When studying records concerned with children, there are a number of familiar words that are used to express the different eras of childhood. These words have always been rather imprecise, which can sometimes make it difficult to interpret what an archive is telling you. 'Baby' can be used to describe children from the time of birth until they are several months old. Parents have generally stopped using the word once their child is able to walk (from 9 months onwards). A baby less than 1 month old is usually called a newborn or, in medical circles, a neonate. Stillbirths or stillborns are babies born dead and usually the cause is not clear although infections are sometimes responsible.

There is some uncertainty about the meaning of the word 'chrisome' when mentioned in connection with a death; it is often said to refer to babies born alive but who died before they were baptised. However, there is no real evidence for this and it more likely refers to babies who died shortly after being baptised – a chrisom being the white robe that a baby was traditionally wrapped in after baptism.

The term 'infant' generally refers to a child aged between a few months old and up to around 3 years of age. A 'youth' was normally what we would today call a teenager, but this word should be interpreted with perhaps more caution then any other described here. There are plenty of quotes from contemporary literature indicating that a youth could be younger than 13 or older than 19:

- 'The other case was a youth aged twenty-one …' – *Cyclopaedia of Practical Medicine*, 1833.
- 'A youth aged twelve took sixty drops …, a youth aged seventeen took forty drops …, a boy aged ten took eight drops …' – *British and Foreign Medical Review*, 1837.
- 'The parents of a youth aged ten years are desirous of placing him under the care of a clergyman …' – *London Review*, 1860.
- 'after one day seeing me conduct a youth aged nine through a quadrille …' – *London Society*, 1865.

Finally, the word 'child' typically describes those who inhabit the intervening years between infant and youth – i.e. around 4 to 12 years of age – but with the same caveats as apply to the word youth above, that it is an inexact term.

Diphtheria

Epidemics of diphtheria have occurred in Europe for at least 2,500 years, and were a major cause of the deaths of children until comparatively recently. In the twentieth century there were often more than 50,000 cases per year in England and Wales until immunisation was introduced.

Diphtheria is caused by infection with bacteria called *Corynebacterium diphtheriae*. It's a contagious disease and spreads from person to person in droplets when people cough or sneeze. Hence it's often associated with crowded, deprived areas where it can spread quickly. In the era before vaccination, children were more vulnerable to diphtheria because adults had been gradually exposed to the bacteria in the environment as they grew up, or had already survived an infection, and as a result had generally became immune to it.

The first signs of diphtheria are typically a fever and sore throat, and this is often followed by a cough. A greyish membrane can grow at the back of the throat and this may block the airway and choke people, hence diphtheria became known as the 'strangling angel of children'. Around 5–10 per cent of sufferers died from the disease and its complications. Diphtheria is commonly found on death certificates from the 1850s to the 1930s because it experienced waves of resurgence during this time. It is sometimes referred to as membranous croup, malignant sore throat, or putrid fever.

JD Brown, a GP, reported the dreadful effects of the 1849–50 diphtheria epidemic in Haverfordwest on local children:

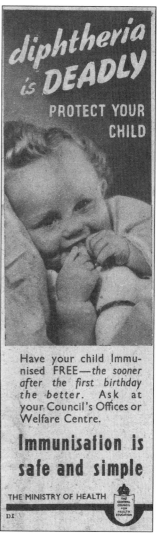

Have your child Immunised FREE—the sooner after the first birthday the better. Ask at your Council's Offices or Welfare Centre.

Immunisation is safe and simple

THE MINISTRY OF HEALTH

An advertisement for the diphtheria vaccination, part of the campaign in the 1940s.

In its course it was very uncertain. Some of the little sufferers appeared to get through easily; others, lingering for weeks with slight but still deceitful symptoms. The child would play almost with every evidence of perfect health, and enjoy the little sports of childhood as usual, when all at once the breathing would become croupy, the inspiration laborious – the pharynx [throat] is attacked! The chances are now fearfully against him. No treatment seems to check it. Time is short, as every minute exhausts life. I have seen them die in four hours after such sudden invasions; they may linger four or six days, with deceitful intermissions of sometimes eight or twelve hours duration. The croupy symptoms would suddenly cease; the little sufferer would sit up, smile, eat, drink, amuse itself; the delighted parents would point to him with admiration of your skill; the sonorous breathing which to you told too plainly, at your last visit, that death was there, has disappeared, and, off your guard, you join in the general joy and stamp it by promising him safe. Mark! Such sudden changes are never to last – it is sure to return. When recovery is to take place, the changes are slow, hesitating, and doubtful for hours and days. Perhaps not more than four hours have passed – you are sent for – the frightful symptoms have returned, generally at night – all now is over; the case is nearly hopeless.

Tragically, although an effective vaccine was available in the 1930s, Britain didn't adopt it and during this decade diphtheria remained the second commonest cause of children dying. The main obstacle seems to have been indecision about who should organise and pay for the immunisation programme. However, the potential dangers posed by a wartime diphtheria epidemic seem to have galvanised the government into action and vaccination was introduced in the 1940s.

In 1943, the last epidemic in Western Europe affected an estimated 1 million people. However, once vaccination was introduced, the number of cases plummeted. In 2010 only eight cases were reported in Britain, and no child has died from diphtheria here since 1982.

Measles
Measles was also known historically as rubeola or morbilli. It is often thought of as a mild disease, but measles can have devastating effects on a population with no immunity to it as native peoples in the Pacific islands discovered to their cost when they first came into contact with it. For example, in 1874, British seamen brought measles to Fiji and it wiped out a third of the population.

Measles is caused by a virus. It starts with symptoms like a cold, and then a fever comes on. After a few days, a classic reddish rash develops on the head then spreads over the rest of the body. Some children get earache, stomach upset, or even fits.

In his *Modern Practice of Physic*, published in 1809, Robert Thomas summed up the main threat posed by measles in Britain: 'The consequences attendant on the measles are frequently more to be dreaded than the immediate disease; for although a person may get through it, and appear for a time to be recovered, still hectic symptoms and pulmonary consumption shall afterwards arise and destroy him.' So it was often the aftermath of measles that killed children – when they were weak they could succumb to chest infections or even meningitis.

Meningitis
The meninges are membranes that surround the brain and spinal cord, and infection with various bacteria or viruses can make them inflamed.

This is meningitis, and it characteristically causes a severe headache, vomiting, and fever, whilst some people go on to develop general aches, a stiff neck, an intolerance of light (photophobia), and a rash. If the infection progresses beyond the initial phase, the victim starts to become drowsy and confused, and may behave strangely. They may also experience fits. Importantly, a proportion of infected people have very vague symptoms that don't entirely fit this 'classic' pattern and they may simply collapse suddenly after feeling unwell for a while.

Bacterial meningitis is much more likely to be fatal than that caused by viruses, but ultimately the mental processes will deteriorate further in many victims, as physician William Gerhard described in the *Medical Examiner*, 1838: 'If, however, the affection should not yield, and passes into the chronic state, the patient remains necessarily more or less insane, and is apt to sink into the third stage of insanity or dementia. He becomes utterly incoherent, and the case usually terminates in a very curious but totally incurable variety of paralysis.'

Symptoms of meningitis in infants and young children are far vaguer than in teenagers which makes it even harder to pick up early.

Mumps

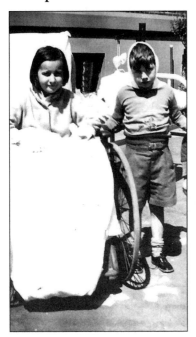

A girl with paralysis due to polio in a wheelchair, and a boy with his face wrapped in a white cloth because of the pain from mumps.

This odd disease is caused by a virus that triggers painful swelling of the glands that produce saliva at the back of the mouth, resulting in a fat 'hamster face' appearance. Sufferers also get a fever, headache, nausea, and flu-like symptoms. Adults and older children may have complications – for example, men may have swelling of the testicles. Mumps has sometimes been called parotitis or cynanche parotidea.

Mumps is rarely fatal and requires little specific treatment, but it is contagious and repeated epidemics have occurred. In the past, a cloth was often tied around the face and knotted at the top to keep the head and face warm, and to offer the tender areas some protection. You may occasionally pick this up in old family photos.

Polio

This condition is more formally termed poliomyelitis, but has also been called infantile paralysis and is caused by a virus. It has always been feared because although most people infected with polio have no symptoms, about 1 per cent of children become paralysed as a result of it. This may explain a disability in your family that you have uncovered during your research.

Ironically, modern sanitation may have been to blame for increasing the rate of polio's paralysing effects. Before there was clean drinking water, babies readily contracted mild polio from contaminated water or from contact with infected persons, and they suffered no ill effects. Sanitation made this early, harmless, contact less common, but when infants or older children are infected they are much more likely to be paralysed. So paralysing forms of polio seem to occur with greater frequency from the late Victorian period until the early 1960s.

The extent of paralysis varied, but it meant a blighted future life for thousands of unfortunate sufferers – leaving the survivors dependent on crutches or wheelchairs in many cases. In their later years, some sufferers experience further deterioration. Unhappily, there are still thousands of men and women living in Britain with paralysis from polio they contracted in the 1950s and 60s.

Polio vaccination was welcomed with an enormous sense of relief in the 1960s. Many of us will remember the polio vaccine as a drop of liquid on a sugar cube: both parents and children alike were often grateful that a needle wasn't required! These days that old vaccine has been replaced by an injection, but immunisation has proved so successful that the World Health Organization (WHO) aims to eradicate polio from the planet using methods similar to those that destroyed smallpox.

Rubella

You should be wary that the word 'rubella' is similar to 'rubeola', an old name for measles. The symptoms of rubella, or 'German measles', can even look like measles because there is a rash, but it is a different disease that was recognised by German doctors first – hence the alternative name. Other symptoms include swollen glands in the neck, fever, and cold-like symptoms.

It's a mild viral disease, but much more serious if it infects a pregnant woman because it can harm the unborn baby. Rubella can make babies deaf, and damage their eyes, hearts, or brains. Protecting babies has thus been the primary motive behind vaccination, which was introduced in the 1970s.

Scarlet Fever

This is caused by an infection with *Streptococcus* bacteria and was also known as scarlatina. It begins with a sore throat, headache, stomach upset, and general aches, and the patient goes on to develop a very red tongue, a characteristic reddish whole-body rash, and a high fever.

The sore throat was the big early warning sign, but we now know that many different bacteria and viruses can cause a sore throat and that scarlet fever itself varies in its severity in individuals: the bacteria causing it can release a poison or toxin that some people react to particularly badly. These differences in patient outcome puzzled many doctors before the twentieth century, and writers frequently remarked upon the greatly varied progress of their patients. They were keen to describe the many different varieties of scarlet fever, the most serious being the 'scarlatina maligna' which was commonly fatal. William Macmichael, who stated 'that the very name of it inspires such dread', also described the worst scarlet fever cases in his *A New View of the Infection of Scarlet Fever*, 1822:

> Ulcers in the throat are visible sometimes on the very first day of the fever; the sores are numerous, deep and sordid. The patient becomes hoarse and almost dumb. Sometimes the whole skin is intensely red at the commencement of the distemper; at other times only the breast and arms have this colour … The condition of the sores is to be considered as indicating the danger of the disease, which must be judged to be greater in proportion as these ulcers occupy a larger space, are deeper, more firmly fixed, and of a more gangrenous hue. In fatal cases the patient becomes, on the second day, comatose, breathes with great difficulty, bending back his head as far as possible. At the same time a purulent and highly offensive matter flows from his nostrils; the throat on inspection is found to be gangrenous and death soon follows.

The children affected were mainly in the age range of 5 to 15 years old, and the infection could spread quickly between people via droplets in exhaled breath and sneezes, so in some situations outbreaks could kill many children quite quickly. In the pre-antibiotic era, this disease killed up to 20 per cent of those with true scarlet fever. They died either from the direct effects of the infection, or because of the ensuing complications such as pneumonia and septicaemia. There are also sometimes long-term after effects such as damage to the kidneys and the heart. When the heart is damaged it can predispose people to heart failure in later life and this was sometimes called rheumatic fever because of a common association with painful joints at the time of the infection. Rheumatic fever can happen even when the original sore throat is quite mild.

Whooping Cough and Croup

The main feature of whooping cough infection is the forceful and severe attacks of coughing it produces. During these attacks, children can only draw breath with difficulty, producing a characteristic 'whoop' noise as they struggle to breathe. The coughing can be so intense that children go blue, vomit, or even faint, and they often become very tired. It has also been known as chink cough, tussis convulsiva, or pertussis.

Around one in every hundred young infants and babies with whooping cough die, sometimes due to its direct effects but also its complications such as pneumonia. It was a common bacterial infection in the past, so even a 1 per cent rate of fatality meant it often killed thousands of children each year. The mortality statistics for 1838, for example, show that 9,107 children died of whooping cough – making it the tenth most common cause of death of people of any age in that year. Vaccination for whooping cough was introduced in the 1950s.

It is possible that some cases diagnosed as whooping cough were due to the infection known as croup, which is usually caused by a virus. Croup involves a swelling of the throat and upper airways so that children experience a barking cough and hoarse voice. The means of differentiating between the two conditions was explained to doctors by Dr Patrick Blair in the eighteenth century, but his means of distinction leaves plenty of room for mis-diagnosis. The following extract is taken from Dr Blair's *Observations in the Practice of Physic*, 1718:

> The tussis convulsiva, or chink-cough, is also some years epidemical and becomes universal among children; as is a certain distemper with us called the Croops – with this variety, that whereas the chink-cough increases gradually, is of long continuance, seizes in paroxysms ['bursts'], and the patient is well in the interval; this convulsion of the larynx [i.e. croup] as it begins so it continues: so violently that unless the child be relieved in a few hours 'tis carried off within twenty-four, or at most, forty-eight hours. When they are seized they have a terrible snorting at the nose and squeaking in the throat, without the least minute of free breathing, and that of a sudden, when perhaps the child was but a little time before healthful and well. The most immediate cure is instant bleeding at the

jugular, either by the lancet or leeches; when the most urgent symptoms are gone, then emetics or the like are administered at discretion.

Other Infections

Children are subject to a large number of additional infections which are often not severe such as chickenpox, mild stomach bugs, and colds. But they are affected by many more serous infections that also affect adults such as chest infections (Chapter 6), bowel infections (Chapter 10), and influenza (Chapter 14). Babies and infants who develop fever as a result of any infection may fit because of their high body temperature, and in this situation death certificates and other sources of information may simply list convulsions, fits, or seizures as the cause of death. This reflects the fact that in former times the precise infection was often not identified.

Nowadays, our children are more protected from infection than at any time in the past thanks to vaccines, antibiotics, clean water, and easy access to healthcare. This is reflected in a vastly reduced mortality rate for children in the modern era, as highlighted in Chapter 1. If our ancestors could speak to us, they would say that's something we should be very grateful for.

Chapter 8

CHOLERA

Cholera is a frightening disease that runs rapidly through a whole community, leaving a trail of bodies in its wake. These days it's usually associated with wars and environmental disasters in third-world countries: for example, there was an outbreak on the island of Haiti after the earthquake there in 2010. The disease is believed to have originated in India, but during the nineteenth century cholera spread speedily to continents as far away as Europe and North America. These Victorian pandemics killed tens of millions of people, and during this time Britain was gripped by cholera four times, although it persisted for longer periods in many other countries.

First Wave

Our nineteenth-century ancestors had to contend with a range of ever-present infections such as TB, but cholera was not native to the British Isles. It was a frightening new invader and by autumn 1831 our ancestors had known it was coming Britain's way for months. British newspapers had recorded the rapid and widespread deaths that marked its trail across Europe from India, and it was simply a matter of time before it reached these shores.

Attempts were made to prevent the arrival of cholera by quarantining ships that came from ports where the disease was known. But in vain. The first fatal case was in Sunderland in October 1831. Just 15 hours after she started vomiting, 12-year old Isabella Hazard died. From this epicentre, cholera spread to seize the nation.

The symptoms were alarming. A few people had mild warning signs, but most were suddenly gripped without warning by dramatic diarrhoea and vomiting. In the severest cases, the loss of body fluids was so appalling that victims rapidly became dehydrated, cold, shrivelled and gaunt. Often their faces were so withered they became almost unrecognisable. Some victims developed a blue-grey skin colour; hence cholera's other name of the 'blue plague'.

Once cholera arrived, local boards of health attempted to limit its spread: initially by trying to isolate confirmed cases, and then by dedicating premises to house the sick. In some parts of the country, such as Liverpool, the population panicked and then rioted – demanding protection. Doctors were even blamed for causing the disease and of using it as a means to obtain bodies for dissection.

One anonymous author recalled the horrors of cholera assaulting a town in northern England in 1832, as published in the *Quarterly Christian Spectator*, 1838:

> The fearful certainty that the cholera was among us struck us with dismay. It was not creeping about with the slow movements of ordinary disease, but with lightning rapidity was leaping from house to house, grappling and crushing its victims like some hideous monster delighting in misery and blood.
>
> Then commenced a scene of panic, at the very recollection of which the mind sickens. Some flying from the city with the seeds of the pestilence in their constitution were taken on the road, and almost literally died by the way-side … Others had recourse to preventive medicines … Still greater numbers had recourse to the brandy bottle to cheer their spirits. All this while the daily numbers of deaths was increasing. It mounted upward from 20 to 50, 80, 100, 150 each twenty-four hours, till it seemed as if our fate were sealed and the curse of heaven was to sweep us all to the grave. When we walked out, the deserted streets, the unfinished buildings abandoned by the workmen, the hearse and dead-carts was frightful … The man whom we met yesterday was today carried to the grave; the person who rose in health was by sunset in his coffin.

Cholera spread quickly and this first wave killed over 32,000 people by the time it petered out here in autumn 1832.

Second Wave

There followed a long lull with no new British cases, but in 1848 cholera returned to wreak its most extensive death toll. In the days before the discovery of bacteria, the most frightening thing about cholera was that no one knew what caused it. To the population at large it looked like a random form of invading death: people seemed to be singled out unpredictably and suddenly, and this added to the fear.

We now know cholera is a waterborne infection that spreads because of poor sanitation. The excrement of people with the disease is laden with

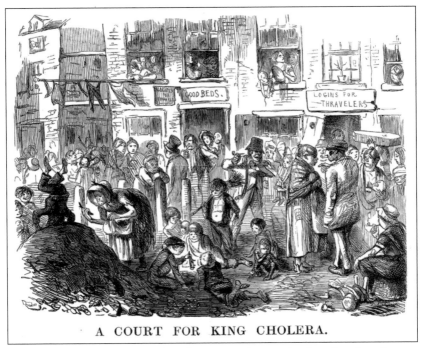

A COURT FOR KING CHOLERA.

This Victorian cartoon shows that cholera was king in the dirty London slums.

bacteria and when this enters the water supply it can then infect everyone who drinks the polluted water. This means that our ancestors living in crowded inner city areas in Britain, where there was limited access to clean water, were particularly likely to be affected.

In the *Morning Chronicle* of 1849, the journalist Henry Mayhew recorded the deplorable state of London's water supply in the slum areas of Bermondsey at the height of the second wave of cholera:

> In this street the cholera first appeared seventeen years ago, and spread up it with fearful virulence; but this year it appeared at the opposite end, and ran down it with like severity. As we passed along the reeking banks of the sewer the sun shone upon a narrow slip of the water. In the bright light it appeared the colour of strong green tea, and positively looked as solid as black marble in the shadow – indeed it was more like watery mud than muddy water; and yet we were assured this was the only water the wretched inhabitants had to drink. As we gazed in horror at it, we saw drains and sewers emptying their filthy contents into it; we saw a whole tier of doorless privies in the

open road, common to men and women, built over it; we heard bucket after bucket of filth splash into it.

And yet, as we stood doubting the fearful statement, we saw a little child lower a tin can with a rope to fill a large bucket that stood beside her. In each of the balconies that hung over the stream the self-same tub was to be seen in which the inhabitants put the mucky liquid to stand, so that they may, after it has rested for a day or two, skim the fluid from the solid particles of filth, pollution, and disease. As the little thing dangled her tin cup as gently as possible into the stream, a bucket of night-soil was poured down from the next gallery.

In this wretched place we were taken to a house where an infant lay dead of the cholera. We asked if they really did drink the water? The answer was, 'They were obliged to'.

People living and working in ports – the main route of entry for the disease – were more prone to cholera than those living in the countryside. Working class urban individuals with roles such as dock worker, servant, tradesman, laundress and so forth were most likely to contract cholera because they were often crowded into areas with a shared water supply. Since wealthy people were more likely to have access to clean water and had proper sanitation, they were least susceptible.

The Victorians recognised that cleanliness was important to prevent disease, but did not understand why. During all the cholera outbreaks doctors did what they could for patients but were hampered principally by a lack of understanding of what caused the disease. It was widely recognised that cholera broke out in dirty places, so people believed that smelly air or 'miasma' caused it. This led to attempts to fumigate affected buildings and ships by burning sulphur and other substances to cleanse them. It was widely believed that drinking brandy prevented the disease.

Yet when the second wave of cholera dissipated in autumn 1849 it left a shocking 52,000 of our ancestors dead.

Third Wave

The movement of European troops during the Crimean War made it impossible to contain a growing spread of cholera, and many British soldiers and seamen abroad were affected in the 1850s. Eventually outbreak number three entered Britain via Newcastle in 1853.

However, once again, after about a year the dread disease died out in the country. But by late 1854 around 20,000 had perished in its wake.

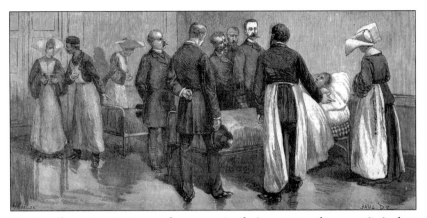

Nineteenth-century doctors gather around a cholera victim; there was little they could do and they often did more harm than good.

Cholera's victims died because of dehydration. Unfortunately, Victorian doctors did little to improve their patients' situation and probably hastened their demise in some cases. Doctors were slaves to their preconceptions about the causes of disease and believed the body needed to be purged of its impurities. So they prescribed potent laxatives, and drugs to make people sick, to patients already exhausted by diarrhoea and vomiting. They administered poisonous mercury – which could cause diarrhoea – and opium which made people vomit; whilst their brandy, bloodletting, and 'hot air baths' made the dehydration worse. Some doctors prescribed even more ludicrous treatments such as highly toxic arsenic. It's a wonder that anyone survived their ministrations. Yet survive they did, and despite shocking symptoms and poor treatment only about 3–4 per cent of people infected with cholera actually died.

However, two doctors eventually did more than anyone else to counteract the threat of cholera by explaining how the disease arose. John Snow proved in 1854 that cholera was spread by contaminated water, and the importance of a clean public water supply was subsequently recognised as vital. Nonetheless, it was not until 1883 that Robert Koch discovered that the disease was caused by a species of bacteria, *Vibrio cholerae*.

Fourth Wave

Cholera's last outing in Britain caused the fewest deaths – a little over 10,000 in total – and it started with a more southerly focus. A small outbreak in Southampton in 1865 was quickly stifled with quarantine

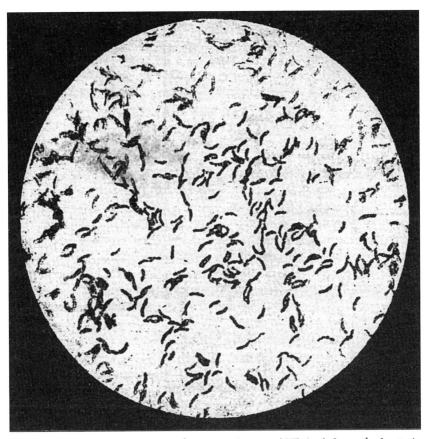

The culprit revealed – a nineteenth-century image of *Vibrio cholerae*, the bacteria that cause cholera.

measures, but a larger wave of disease in 1866 killed nearly 5,000 people in London, mainly in the East End. Other areas where large numbers of people suffered in this outbreak were the north-west of England (where over 2,000 died), Wales, and the south-east of England.

This last wave did a great deal to drive forward improved sanitation in Britain.

Your Ancestors and Cholera

On death certificates, this disease is usually termed simply 'cholera', but it was also known as cholera morbus, and Asiatic, pestilential, or epidemic cholera. Confusingly, before the advent of the pandemics, the term 'cholera' had previously been used to describe mild disorders like gastroenteritis. Some doctors started to call this 'English cholera' or 'cholera nostras' instead.

In Britain, cholera arrived, ran its course for about a year, and then disappeared again. This means that all cases of cholera found on death certificates in Britain are confined to the same years: 1831–2, 1848–9, 1853–4, and 1865–6.

Yet cholera also affected British people abroad – particularly men serving with the army in the Crimea, merchant seamen and their passengers visiting affected ports, and people working in cholera's epicentre of India. In these cases, the deaths occurred over a much wider spread of years.

It's quite common to find cholera cited on British memorial plaques dedicated to ancestors who died abroad. An example in Holy Trinity Church, Gosport, commemorates William Rogers 'commander of the ship *Startled Fawn* of Liverpool who fell a victim to cholera while in the zealous charge of his duties at Calcutta, 28th June 1858'.

Impressed with the disastrous novelty of cholera, and keen to share their experiences, many doctors wrote up their cases in medical journals in an era when patient confidentiality was not considered important. Thus many journals carry details of the deaths of named individuals. A particularly good example is the *Cholera Gazette* of 1832, available on Google Books at http://books.google.com.

Ignorance of the causes of the disease led many communities to establish separate cholera graveyards for victims, in an attempt to isolate the disease. Some of these still survive such as the Cholera Burial Ground in York. However, during the outbreaks many victims were hastily buried without an individual memorial stone, and many of the burial grounds are now lost.

Twenty-first Century

The WHO provides information on the modern management of cholera, www.who.int/topics/cholera/en/. Mercifully, greater understanding of the disease means that pandemics of cholera no longer seem to occur, but in 2010 the WHO still estimated that up to 120,000 people die from it every year around the world.

Chapter 9

DIET AND STARVATION

What we eat or drink can have a profound effect on our health. For example, contaminated food and water can transmit disease and cause infections such as dysentery (see Chapter 10), a poor diet can increase the risk of heart disease (Chapter 13), and the deleterious effects of chronic heavy alcohol intake are discussed in Chapter 4.

But health is also obviously affected by ingesting too little food (or too much), by a diet that lacks key nutritional elements, and by inadvertently eating food containing poisons.

Starvation

From the relative comfort of the twenty-first century, it can be hard to believe that Britain has suffered from famine – widespread prolonged starvation leading to the deaths of its citizens. However, this has happened on many occasions in the past 2,000 years. Earlier societies were heavily dependent on locally grown crops, and before 1800 few foodstuffs were imported except for luxury items such as spices, spirits and wine, tea and coffee. The country depended for its survival largely on what its own population could grow. This was a not unreasonable expectation because the population was considerably smaller than it is now.

Yet the margin of security in this arrangement was relatively small. Storage facilities were primitive and people relied on eating what was 'in season', so in the event of a disaster there was little back-up. And disasters did happen. What if there was widespread crop failure due to the weather? What if disease or war meant there were not enough people to plant or harvest the crops?

In the Middle Ages there were many famines that affected all or parts of the country. In the thirteenth century alone there were twenty-two. In 1235, for example, a famine in the wake of war, plague, and persistent bad weather killed 20,000 people in London alone. People were reduced to eating tree bark, horses, grass, and whatever else they could lay their hands upon. Not surprisingly, this situation improved only slowly, for in the following year it is recorded in John Stow's *A Survay of London* that:

> William de Haverhill, the king's treasurer, was commanded that upon the day of the circumcision of our Lord that 6,000 poor people should be fed at Westminster … The like commandment the said King Henry gave to Hugh Gifford and William Brown that upon Friday next, after the Epiphany, they should cause to be fed in the great hall at Windsor at a good fire, all the poor and needy children that could be found. [1598 edition.]

In 1258, the contemporary chronicler Matthew Paris in his *Historia Anglorum* describes the effects of yet another famine:

> About the same time, such great famine and mortality prevailed in the country, that a measure of wheat rose in price to fifteen shillings and more, at a time when the country itself was drained of money, and numberless dead bodies were lying about the streets. No one, indeed, could remember ever having before beheld such misery and such famine, although there were many who had seen prices rise higher than they now were. Unless corn had been brought for sale from the continent, the rich would scarcely have been able to escape death. Moreover, the dead lay about, swollen up and rotting, on dunghills, and in the dirt of the streets, and there was scarcely any one to bury them; nor did the citizens dare or choose to receive the dead into their houses, for fear of contagion.

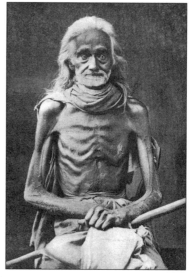

Extreme starvation produces loss of body fat and muscle wasting; victims become weak, apathetic, and are prone to infection.

During a famine people literally starved to death or were so weakened by lack of food that they succumbed to infection, or even committed suicide. Even when they didn't die, malnutrition produced vitamin deficiencies that could lead to other medical problems, and in children to impaired growth and development.

Examples of Famines

It would not be possible to itemise every famine that has afflicted Britain because there have been far too many, but some significant examples from the past 500 years are given below.

1586–7

There were many episodes of famine in sixteenth-century Britain. The poor lived principally on barley and so when grain harvests failed, the vast majority of the population was affected. A couple of severe winters and two very dry summers produced poor harvests (a 'dearth') and culminated in famine all over Europe in 1586, with recurrences in the 1590s. The north of England was hit particularly hard as can be seen from death rates in many parish registers. The famines of late Elizabethan England helped to usher in more formal Poor Laws which aimed to protect those in each parish who were genuinely suffering. Local Overseers of the Poor knew the people in their community who were in real need – such as the sick, the elderly, and orphans – and were tasked to provide for them. The so-called 'idle poor' or 'sturdy beggars', on the other hand, were not supported.

1649

A famine ensued in Lancashire and the northern counties of England 'occasioned by the frequent ravages, marches and spoils' of soldiers in the Civil War.

1690s

Scotland experienced a famine that led to a drop in the population of around 15 per cent during this decade; in areas of the Highlands the figure may have exceeded 20 per cent. Erratic weather during the growing seasons led to a succession of disastrous harvests for grain and other commodities. There were attempts to import grain but this was not very successful because of the poor harvests in many other European countries. The population declined because of death from starvation and a reduced birth rate, but also – for perhaps the first time in a British famine – due to emigration: many Scots fled to Ireland.

1727–8

Some parts of the Midlands were affected by famine when a poor harvest occurred in the midst of typhus and typhoid outbreaks.

1740–1

The Irish Famine was caused by a long cold and dry period that resulted in successive poor harvests. There were food riots as staple products like potatoes and oats became short in supply, and prices rose. Many poor families starved to death.

1816

In the wake of the disruption brought about by the Napoleonic Wars, and a series of poor domestic harvests, a massive eruption of Mount Tambora in Indonesia seems to have triggered a near-global climate change for a year or more. This brought unseasonably cold temperatures, not conducive to growing crops. The peculiar prevailing climate led 1816 to be dubbed the 'Year Without a Summer', and it worsened an already precarious situation so that food came into short supply, and soup kitchens had to be set up around the country. In some cities, such as Glasgow and Dundee, there were food riots.

1845–52

Two famines happened simultaneously – the Great Famine (or Potato Famine) in Ireland and the Highland Potato Famine in Scotland. In both areas, farmers grew potatoes as the most rewarding crop, and the population depended upon it to feed their families. When the potatoes were struck by a disease called potato blight, the harvest failed on a monumental scale depriving the people of a staple part of their diet.

The situation in Ireland rapidly deteriorated – there was mass starvation, and the inept or uncaring British government did little to help. Around 1 million people died of disease and malnutrition, whilst a similar number emigrated to the USA, Canada, Australia, and England. Scottish men and women emigrated too.

In *Transactions of the Central Relief Committee During the Famine in Ireland 1846 and 1847*, John Crossfield reported to the Quakers attempting to provide some relief in Ireland that:

In many cases whole families were swept away by starvation, fever, or both. In one cabin I saw six children lying heads and points on their miserable beds on each side of the turf fire, while the father and mother, wasted and emaciated, sat crouching over the embers. In another cabin I saw the father lying near the point of death on one side of the fireplace; over the ashes sat a wretched little boy, wholly naked – and on the opposite side of the hut, beneath a ragged quilt, lay the body of an old woman who had taken shelter there and died. As she belonged to nobody, there was nobody to bury her, and there have been many instances of bodies lying five or six days unburried.

The shadowy figure of death tries to urge the wealthy and privileged to wake up to the potato famine in Ireland.

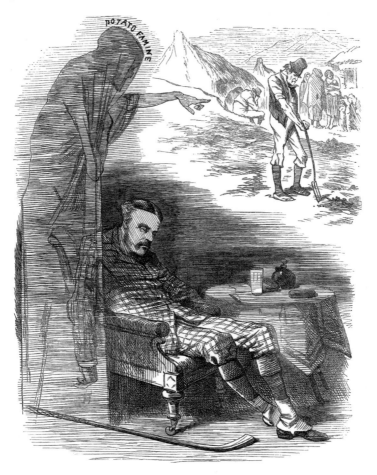

1879

A 'mini famine' in Ireland caused widespread hunger, but few deaths compared to the Great Famine of thirty years before.

Even when there was no famine, individual families or communities might starve and survive at close to subsistence level due to economic hardship. In Victorian times, despite revision of the Poor Laws in 1834, the care of the vulnerable and the management of workhouses were often shockingly inhumane. Destitute and seriously ill individuals could be pushed from pillar to post because no one wanted to pay for their care. The hard-hearted attitude to poverty displayed by some Victorians is not just a fiction created by writers like Dickens – it really did happen. For example, the *Champion and Weekly Herald* from 1838 reports this typical case (edited):

DEATH BY STARVATION
An inquest was held before Mr E D Conyers on Wednesday, on the body of Elizabeth Lyon, which was lying at the union workhouse, Great Driffield, Yorkshire. After the jury had been sworn, they proceeded to view the body, which presented a dreadfully emaciated appearance, being nothing but skin and bone. It appeared from the evidence produced, that the deceased was unmarried, and 40 years of age; that she had resided at Bridlington for a long time, was of a loose character, having had several illegitimate children, one of which, a boy of ten years of age is still living, and that she belonged to the parish of Kelk, in the Driffield Union, from which parish she had no out-door relief.

Mr Henry Grozier, the relieving officer of the Driffield union, said that he received the deceased on the 30th of April, that when she got into the workhouse she was so weak as not to be able to speak for some time. He asked her why she did not apply to the Bridlington Union for relief. She said she had done so, but that they would not give her any thing, and that she had been hungered and starved to death.

David Whiting, relieving officer of the Bridlington Union, said that neither the deceased nor any one for her applied to him for relief; if she had, he would have supplied her.

Dinah Coatham, of Bridlington, said she had known Elizabeth Lyon from childhood. She recollected, at the request of the deceased, going to David Whiting the relieving officer at

Bridlington, about three or four weeks ago, to ask him for relief for Elizabeth Lyon; she asked for 1 shilling, and he said he would not give her anything.

The jury after a patient investigation of the whole of the circumstances, returned the following verdict:

> 'That Elizabeth Lyon departed this life by the visitation of God in a natural way, and that the jurors do further say that the death of Elizabeth Lyon has been accelerated by want of the necessaries of life and medicine, and that considerable blame attaches to David Whiting, the relieving officer at Bridlington, for not having paid proper attention to the application of the said Elizabeth Lyon for relief.'

Mr Whiting escaped prosecution. In Victorian times, public officials in similar positions were repeatedly and consistently allowed to evade their responsibility for having allowed fellow human beings to die. Many paupers – as they were then called – starved to death. Something that was typically described as 'want of the necessities of life', as it was in the case of poor Elizabeth Lyon. Emaciation and wasting away due to starvation is often called marasmus on death certificates.

Workhouses could, and did, close their doors to people dying of hunger. This building is now a hospital but was originally the South Stoneham Union Workhouse in Hampshire.

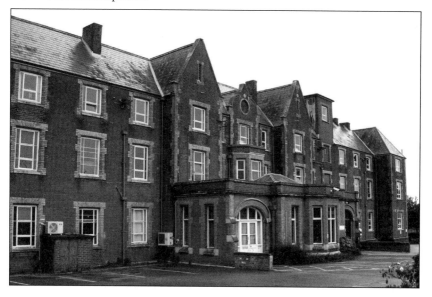

Deficient Diets

In any situation where food is in short supply, or where choice is limited, then it is possible that the resulting unbalanced diet will lead to deficiencies of vitamins or minerals. Historically, scurvy – caused by a lack of vitamin C – has been the biggest killer (see Chapter 19).

However, there are other important examples. Deficiency of vitamin D in childhood leads to rickets, also known as rachitis, a disease where bones do not form properly. Victims suffer from pain in their bones, feel weak, and are much more prone to fractures. They often develop abnormally shaped bones because lack of vitamin D makes them soft. The classic examples are being bow-legged, a deformity that can be quite dramatic, and also a bent spine and changes to the shape of the skull.

In adults, vitamin D deficiency is called osteomalacia, although in former times it was sometimes called malacosteon or mollities ossium. As is the case with rickets, those affected with osteomalacia suffer from more frequent bone fractures, weakness, and pain in the bones. Deformities due to lack of vitamin D can affect the shape of the bones surrounding the birth canal in women, and this was sometimes the cause of death in childbirth in former times (see Chapter 18).

Various other illnesses are caused by a lack of specific nutrients. For example, anaemia can be caused by an absence of vitamin B12, folic acid, or iron in the diet.

Some deficiencies can be quite geographically specific. In parts of the Midlands, for example, there is a lack of iodine in the soil. Insufficient iodine stops the human thyroid gland from working and it reacts by swelling up under the chin to form a large protuberance called a goitre. The condition 'Derbyshire Neck' was well known up until the early twentieth century, and adults with the condition tended to be slow in movement and thought. A poorly functioning thyroid during pregnancy also produces babies suffering from a mental retardation formerly known as cretinism.

Another geographically related example is deficiency of vitamin B3 (niacin). This has been common in countries where the population relied on maize or white rice as a staple food. Lack of vitamin B3 causes a multi-symptom disorder known as pellagra.

Poisons in Food

All sorts of substances that can harm people can get into food and drinks, not least the micro-organisms that cause various infections. Some poisons in food arise from toxins that bacteria produce. Botulism is the most famous of these – causing paralysis that can prove fatal when *Clostridium botulinum* bacteria are allowed to grow in food that is not cooked properly before eating. Interestingly, the potent toxin that these bacteria produce is now used cosmetically in very small doses to treat facial ageing because it paralyses the muscles that produce wrinkles (e.g. Botox).

However, other poisons are not connected to microorganisms at all. Lead is a good example, which has been a persistent offender throughout history in various guises. People with lead poisoning often have very severe bowel pains or colic, start to behave oddly, and may fit and even die. This condition is also known as plumbism, saturnism, or colica pictonum. Yet lead pipes transported drinking water for centuries, lead-containing vessels were used to store or cook food, and lead-based chemicals were added to foods and drinks to improve flavour by making them sweeter and less acidic. In an appendix to his *Essay on the Liverpool Spa Water*, Dr Thomas Houlston writing in 1773 noted that adding lead to foods, or cooking or storing food in lead containers, had 'repeatedly proved fatal'. He goes on to relate the following anecdote:

> In the late Duke of Newcastle's family, when at Hanover in June 1752, thirty two persons were seiz'd with the metallic colic, after having drank a small white wine adulterated with lead. One of them died epileptic in less than a fortnight, the rest, after suffering much and relapsing frequently, recover'd, except one who remains paralytic.

In south-west England, cider was traditionally made using lead containers up until the second half of the eighteenth century. Cider drinking was associated with an illness called Devonshire colic which was related to some fatalities. This was entirely due to lead poisoning which came about because the acidic apple juice dissolved the lead. Thankfully, the practice of using lead had been phased out by the late 1700s.

Some poisons in food have bizarre origins. The liver of some mammals such as the seal and polar bear contain such high concentrations of vitamin A that it is toxic to humans, as some Arctic explorers discovered to their cost. Ergotism, or St Anthony's fire, is a disease caused by a fungus that grows on cereal crops such as rye. When people eat enough of this contaminant it produces vomiting, fitting, dramatic hallucinations, and gangrene of the fingers and toes. There were periodic outbreaks of this condition in Europe when suitable weather conditions encouraged widespread growth of the fungus.

Chapter 10

DYSENTERY AND BOWEL INFECTIONS

One of the more famously unusual deaths in English history is Henry I's demise due to a 'surfeit of lampreys'. The lamprey is a fish, a common cause of food poisoning, and so a bowel infection was really the most likely reason for his death. Henry I was not the only medieval monarch to die in this way: the notorious King John also succumbed – although his relentless bowel complaint has often been blamed not on lampreys but on peaches. Henry V's death has also been attributed to dysentery. The deaths of three kings illustrates that even at the highest levels of medieval society no one was spared the risk of bowel infections even though the King would receive only the best quality food and drink, and had servants to prepare and serve it. If the most senior person in the country could die from a gut infection, these illnesses must have been common.

Even today, when we understand that bacteria cause disease and can use antibiotics to kill them, people still die from food poisoning. From time to time we hear on the news about victims of some of the more famous bacteria such as *E. Coli* and *Salmonella*. However, deaths in the modern era are on a very much smaller scale than in the past.

Infections of the gut take a variety of forms and different types of micro-organism can be responsible. Cholera is a notable example, which is the subject of Chapter 8 in this book, but there are many others.

Dysentery

The words 'flux', or 'bloody flux', were used in former times to indicate persistent severe diarrhoea. This is usually interpreted as the more modern term 'dysentery'. There are two major types. Bacterial or bacillary dysentery is a bowel infection classically caused by *Shigella* bacteria, but also attributable to other organisms. The second type is amoebic dysentery, which is an infection by various species of single-celled organisms called amoebae. Bacterial dysentery is much more common in Europe, whereas amoebic dysentery is associated with the tropics. Both types occur with greater frequency in hot weather.

Dysentery varies in its severity and many people do recover, but the diarrhoea is typically of prolonged duration. Quite commonly, victims pass liquid stools to start with, and then mucous once the bowel is empty because the bowel lining becomes inflamed and it may even ulcerate. Victims can feel compelled to continue to strain painfully at the lavatory even when there is nothing left to come out. The stools and mucous are often stained with blood, but the blood loss is not in itself serious. There is often abdominal pain, which can be severe and comes in bursts, and sometimes fever, nausea, and vomiting. Symptoms can last many days, and victims may become weak, very cold, and perhaps delirious. Those who die usually do so because they have become too dehydrated.

Individuals are infected when they consume water or food contaminated with bacteria from the faeces of an existing victim. This can easily happen if victims do not wash their hands after going to the lavatory, if toilet facilities are not properly segregated from living quarters, or if the water supply as a whole becomes contaminated. Infected persons can continue to shed bacteria in their faeces for some time after their recovery.

In former times the terms 'dysentery' or 'flux' were probably used to describe a whole range of diarrhoeas caused by infection. This might include often milder conditions that we might call today 'food poisoning' – a term coined in the twentieth century to describe an infection caused by contaminated food regardless of the micro-organism responsible. Before pasteurisation was introduced as a form of sterilisation, infected milk was a particularly common source of the *Shigella* bacteria which cause classic dysentery.

Until micro-organisms had been revealed as the cause of dysentery in the late nineteenth century, the condition was treated using the prevailing medicines of the time. In the seventeenth and eighteenth centuries, doctors believed that since the body was obviously trying to evacuate some noxious substance from the body they would help it do so by bloodletting, administering laxatives such as rhubarb, and using drugs to make the patient vomit such as ipecacuanha. Needless to say, these measures undoubtedly made patients worse by hastening their dehydration. Some doctors dwelled endlessly on the minutiae of the treatment regimen such as whether the rhubarb should be toasted or not before administration to the patient. By the nineteenth century, in a reversal of thinking, doctors were beginning to administer opium, mercury, lead, and other treatments to stop the flood of diarrhoea. Sulphuric acid became a popular treatment – presumably in an attempt to 'normalise' the known acidity of the stomach.

Dysentery at sea was a particular menace, with contaminated food and water supplies on board often being the cause of the illness. The disease was difficult to manage and impossible to contain in such a confined space. In 1811, the surgeon Robert Robertson vividly conjures up the appearance of an affected ship in his *Synopsis Morborum*:

> Of all the diseases which attack a ship's company, the dysentery, if not the most fateful, is, in my opinion, equally so with any other; and by far the most loathsome. The constant doleful complaints from the various violent pains, from gripes, and tenesmus [painful straining]; the continual noxious fetor [smell] about the sick, as well as of the necessary buckets; not to mention how extremely disgusting to the sight such objects must be, in spite of all means which can be used, are evils peculiar to dysentery alone. Yet, great as they are, they are undoubtedly much increased when the weather is so bad as not to admit the lower deck ports to be up in large ships, or the hatch-ways in small ships to be unlayed. The foul air, then being much more confined around the sick and where the well people lie, is consequently drawn into the lungs again and again by respiration, and soon becomes more foul and noxious, which renders it unfit for the salutary purposes of both the sick and the healthy.

Famously, Sir Francis Drake died of dysentery on the *Defiance* in 1596, but whole ships could be disabled by the illness with barely enough crew fit to work the vessel. It could be a frightening time for passengers too, and emigrants packed into ships for long journeys were particularly susceptible.

Another important environment in which dysentery has occurred for many centuries is the army, where it was sometimes referred to as 'campaign fever'. Large numbers of men in close quarters, sharing the same food, water, and toilet facilities enabled disease to spread quickly. It has been estimated that eight times more men died from disease than from fighting during the Napoleonic Wars (1803–15), and dysentery was a major component of this statistic.

Deaths from dysentery in the army should have been preventable. As early as the 1750s, John Pringle, Physician-General to the Army, thought so. He realised that dysentery was 'evidently communicated by the faeces of those who are ill of the distemper'. He thus advocated that soldiers dig latrines deeply, create fresh ones regularly, and that individuals be punished for soiling the ground of the camp instead of using the appointed toilets. He urged commanders not to camp on marshy ground where the water could become stagnant. Pringle's advice, as described in his *Observations on the Diseases of the Army*, 1753, was that: 'Whenever the bloody flux begins to spread, the best means of preservation are to leave the ground, with the privies, foul straw, and other filth of the camp behind: which method is to be repeated once or twice more or oftener, if consistent with the military operations.' He realised that men had to be separated from the source of contamination, including their own effluent, so he also recommended that serious cases be removed from the camp but without congregating all the ill persons together as this could act as a focus for further outbreaks. This was all very sensible, and borne solely from his practical observation of the disease in the field, but these simple hygienic precepts were, sadly, not always adhered to.

Hence we find, over a hundred years later, in the Crimea, dysentery was still a big problem for the armed forces. Thomas Burgess, an army doctor from the Portsmouth Military Hospital, described the effects of dysentery on the war's young soldiers in the *Lancet*, 1856: 'Boys of eighteen wore the haggard time-worn aspect of men of seventy or eighty, with sunken glazed eyes, prominent jaws, and an expression of utter prostration, painful to look at. Their bodies were crawling with vermin and the skin encrusted with filth, and even human excrement.'

Dysentery occurred widely in the unsanitary trenches of the First World War, as well as in various arenas of the Second World War including prison camps. The German field marshal, Rommel, declared that the Battle of El Alamein in 1942 had been a victory for dysentery rather than the British Eighth Army, because around half of his troops had been disabled by the disease.

However, outside the peculiar setting of war, outbreaks of dysentery became increasingly rare after 1800 due to the general improvement in public sanitary conditions and hygiene in Britain. Such outbreaks that did occur tended to be confined to crowded establishments where it could spread quickly such as asylums, prisons, and barracks.

Typhoid

Typhoid is effectively a special kind of dysentery, in that it is a bowel infection caused by bacteria known historically as *Salmonella typhi*. These bacteria are interesting in that they only infect humans and are not known to cause disease in other mammals.

Probably the most famous British victim of typhoid was Queen Victoria's husband, Prince Albert, who died of the illness in 1861. His son, the future Edward VII, contracted the disease but recovered. Another famous sufferer was the Irish woman Mary Mallon, who survived the infection but became a long-term carrier of the disease, infecting over fifty victims after she emigrated to the USA where she worked as a cook. She came known as the infamous 'Typhoid Mary', and had to be incarcerated to stop her continuing to transmit the disease to others.

Typhoid spreads in the same way as other forms of dysentery, but when contaminating food *Salmonella* is particularly prone to growing in dairy products, shellfish and certain meats. The symptoms are similar to dysentery and can persist for weeks, but there is usually a high fever, an abdominal rash, and delirium is common. Victims have a vacant stare said to be characteristic, and are trembly. In children particularly, the infection can damage the kidneys, liver, or brain.

Typhoid has been known by a variety of other names in the past, including enteric fever, gastric fever, pythogenic fever, and nervous fever. It was also somewhat confusingly called abdominal typhus, which has probably helped to perpetuate confusion about the difference between these two unrelated illnesses (see Chapter 23).

William Budd, a physician at Bristol Royal Infirmary, offered a valuable insight into mid-Victorian sanitation and the mechanism by which typhoid spread in the population. In a paper in the *Lancet* in 1856 he re-affirmed Pringle's observations of a century before about dysentery in general: that infected faeces were a source of typhoid infection. Budd remarked that the wealthy were more careful about cleanliness so they were less likely to contract the infection or spread it, but he continues:

> Amongst the poor, such refinements are never thought of; and when this fever breaks out in a poor family, the discharges from the bowels are thrown, without preparation, either into the common privy, or, as I have seen a hundred times in rural districts, are cast upon the dungheap or into the open gutter. From this point, following the line of the watershed, this pestilent stuff often makes its way to considerable distances, where ... it may carry disease and death into many an unsuspecting household.

A vaccine against typhoid was first developed by Almroth Wright in 1896, and immunisation was subsequently given to British troops during the First World War. However, this vaccine only protected against typhoid

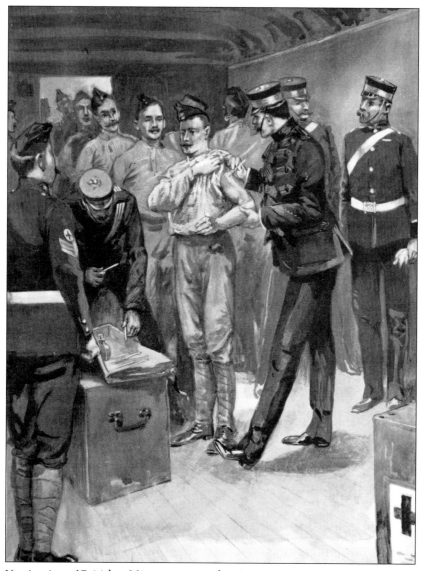

Vaccination of British soldiers against typhoid in 1899.

and not other forms of dysentery. A typhoid vaccine is still recommended for British travellers journeying to certain parts of the world on holiday.

Griping of the Guts

This catch-all phrase is commonly used in the Bills of Mortality of seventeenth and eighteenth-century England to refer to any painful gut disorder, but it accurately reflects the fact that many of our ancestors died because of abdominal pain without the cause being established. We might speculate that causes could include conditions such as bowel cancer (Chapter 5), pancreatitis, dysentery, constipation, and ulcers.

Stomach and intestinal ulcers ('peptic ulcers') are easily healed today with medication, but in the past sufferers could only rely upon modifying their diet to ease the pain. The ulcers frequently worsened over time and if the ulcer burst people died due to internal bleeding, or an abdominal infection called peritonitis when their bowel contents spilled out through the hole in their intestines. This was probably the cause of death of silent-movie idol Rudolph Valentino in 1926. Only in the late twentieth century was it discovered that antibiotics are an important part of the treatment of ulcers because infection with bacteria called *Helicobacter* is commonly the cause.

However, perhaps the most famous cause of abdominal pain is appendicitis. The appendix is a 'blind alley' in the human intestines with a narrow exit so it is inclined to be blocked by hard, undigested items that people gulp down such as pips, fruit stones, and nuts. Children are susceptible because they sometimes swallow small parts of toys, pins, stones or similar items and these can also block the appendix. Once the appendix is blocked it can become infected, ulcerate and then burst. This leads to great pain in the lower right belly near the groin and once the appendix has ruptured the victim dies quickly, usually from peritonitis. The only remedy is an operation to cut out the appendix and stitch up the resulting hole in the gut. This is usually successful if it takes place before the appendix bursts.

The surgeon John Parkinson wrote a classic description of appendicitis which appeared in the *Transactions of the Medical and Chirurgical Society of London* in 1812. In this description, the appendix is termed 'appendix vermiformis', and the 'caecum' that he refers to is the beginning of the large intestine that it joins.

> A preparation of diseased appendix vermiformis in my possession, was removed from a boy about five years of age, who died under the following circumstances.
>
> He had been observed for some time to decline in health, but made no particular complaint until two days before his death, when he was suddenly seized with vomiting, and great prostration of strength. The abdomen became very tumid [swollen] and painful upon being pressed: his countenance pale and sunken, and his pulse hardly perceptible. Death, preceded by extreme restlessness and delirium, took place within twenty-four hours.

... The viscera, independent of the inflammation of their peritoneal covering, appeared in a perfectly healthy state, excepting the appendix vermiformis of the caecum. No diseased appearance was seen in this part near to the caecum; but about an inch of its extremity was considerably enlarged and thickened, its internal surface ulcerated, and an opening from ulceration, which would have admitted a crow-quill, was found at the commencement of the diseased part, about the middle of the appendix, through which it appeared that a thin, dark-coloured, and highly fetid [foul-smelling] fluid, had escaped into the cavity of the abdomen.

Upon opening the appendix, a piece of hardened faeces was found impacted in that part of it which lay between the opening, and that portion of the appendix, which was not evidently marked by disease.

The nineteenth century was a great era for collectors of all kinds and note that Parkinson, like many other doctors of the time, simply kept parts of their ex-patients if they demonstrated something interesting.

In June 1902, after much preparation, the world eagerly anticipated the crowning of a new British King. Yet, rather inconveniently, the unlucky Edward VII, whom we have already noted survived a bout of typhoid as a young man, went down with appendicitis just before the event. He developed peritonitis and was told he must undergo an operation or die. The procedure, however, was successful and the coronation eventually took place in August of that year.

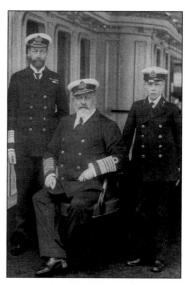

Edward VII (seated, centre) survived life-threatening attacks of typhoid in 1870 and appendicitis in 1902.

Chapter 11

EPILEPSY AND STROKES

Our ancestors were deeply suspicious – even frightened of – diseases that affected the brain. Mental illness is discussed in Chapter 15, but physical diseases that emanated from the brain could also be viewed with some prejudice. A person falling to the ground and fitting might be possessed by an evil spirit, whereas a stroke was maybe the judgement of heaven. Indeed, sudden deaths, such as those that may occur due to a stroke, were often described as the visitation of God until well into the Victorian age.

Doctors didn't know what caused epilepsy or strokes, and some thought that they were related disorders. In the following eighteenth-century advertisement, which appeared in the *Coventry Mercury* in 1761, epilepsy and strokes are conflated with a range of other 'nervous' disorders that made people collapse:

> Dr Lowther's Specific Powders and Drops, have incontestably proved their greatly superior efficacy to the common practice, or any discovery yet made, in the radical cure of all and every species of fits, whether epileptic, convulsive, hysteric, hypochondriac, or paralytic. In fact, they are an absolute cure for the whole train of nervous disorders, with all their concomitant symptoms. Twelve years' experience with uncommon success, confirms their not only curing, but being a most certain preservative against apoplexies, are perfectly innocent, and may be taken by either sex, at all times, and infants. Some thousands have been restored to health by them since their first publication, great numbers of whom were before deemed incurable. The yet incredulous may be referred to, and have the attestations of, more than 500 persons of distinction, who have experienced their salutary effects, after they had very ineffectually tried the whole tribe of other nervous medicines, spa waters, baths, etc. [Modernised spellings and punctuation.]

Epilepsy

Also known since antiquity as the 'falling sickness', epilepsy is famously believed to have afflicted Julius Caesar. The fits that ensue during an acute attack of epilepsy have been variously known as seizures or convulsions. Although note that 'seizure' has been used more generally to refer to short periods of intense medical symptoms in other situations. A patient might suffer a coughing 'seizure', and the term apoplectic 'seizure' implies that apoplexy has gripped the patient not that there has necessarily been fitting.

Fitting can happen spontaneously for no outward reason or trigger, yet it can occur from a variety of definite causes as well, including head injuries (after accidents), during infections that cause fever (especially in infants), as a

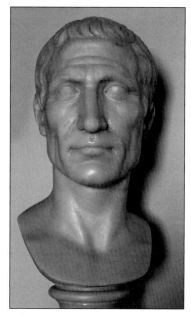

Julius Caesar famously suffered from 'the falling sickness'.

consequence of strokes, and as a feature of alcoholism. The classic fit – or 'tonic-clonic convulsion' – involves the unfortunate sufferer collapsing to the ground; then, as his or her muscles expand and contract, so the person twitches and jerks for a period of time before the convulsion subsides and the patient comes around. There are, however, other kinds of epilepsy where this kind of 'classic' fitting does not happen.

By the early nineteenth century doctors grasped that fits were caused by some sort of structural change in the brain, but despite this realisation they still had some curious notions about the factors that could trigger a fit, including tapeworms, constipation, seeing another patient with epilepsy, fear, masturbating, and particular smells or even colours.

Since the earliest writings about epilepsy, it has been advised that apart from protecting the patient from self-injury there was little to be done to treat a fit. Various means were used to try and prevent fits recurring such as bleeding the patient and 'cures' such as castor oil, copper, iron, and even arsenic. As usual, there were plenty of people prepared to swear by these remedies, but fitting can go away without treatment or be absent for a long time before recurring. However, John Eberle, a nineteenth-century doctor who treated a patient with epilepsy, was honest enough to admit in his *A Treatise on the Practice of Medicine*, 1830:

> [In epilepsy] we are seldom enabled to prescribe with any
> degree of reliance upon general and rational therapeutic
> principles. In this state of perplexity and uncertainty, we have
> often no other alternative left to us than to administer remedies
> without being able to give any other reason for their use than
> that they have occasionally been successfully employed.

The first drug to prevent fits with apparently reasonable success was bromide in the mid-Victorian era, but it was quite toxic and so its use was limited. Barbiturates in the early twentieth century offered a more effective and safer option. From the mid-twentieth century onwards a wider range of effective and safer medicines became available to both alleviate fitting and to prevent fits occurring.

Strokes

Strokes are often called cerebrovascular accidents by doctors these days, but they were described in various ways historically such as 'effusion on the brain'. The word apoplexy is sometimes assumed to mean a stroke. It was undoubtedly used to describe strokes – sometimes called apoplectic seizures – but 'apoplexy' was also used to describe any form of sudden death where the victim was dramatically struck down, i.e. he or she collapsed and died speedily without gaining full consciousness. Large strokes can kill a person swiftly and unexpectedly, but other causes of 'sudden death' that might historically have been called apoplexy include a heart attack, a burst artery (aneurysm), a clot in the lung (pulmonary embolism), or a faulty heart beat (arrhythmia), although strokes and heart attacks are by far the most common causes in the modern world.

The association of apoplexy with some sort of divine retribution – being struck down by God – was in part influenced by the observation that sudden collapses were more likely when an older person became very angry, had sex, or over-ate – behaviour related to the sins of anger, lust, and gluttony. Yet one suspects that a large number of these sudden deaths – whether labelled as apoplexy or not – were due to heart attacks (see Chapter 13).

Patients were also described in terms of the effects of their stroke. A 'palsy' referred to a distinct part of the body that was paralysed (e.g. one half of the face, or one arm). The more general terms 'paralysis', 'paresis', or 'weakness' were applied to affected stroke victims and tended to imply a hierarchy of loss of function, with paralysis being the most severe. But note that paralysis can also be caused by, for example, accidents, polio, meningitis, syphilis etc.

Doctors tried to identify the causes of stroke by contemplating causative factors. Curiously, they seemed to have focused quite a lot on the gut as a culprit – flatulence and constipation being widely regarded as dangerous by nineteenth-century doctors – together with those twin Victorian evils of 'immoderate living' and 'excitement'.

Apart from general supportive care, there was little that could be done for stroke victims who survived, until well into the twentieth century. Daniel MacLachan noted of stroke survivors in 1863 that 'although life may be preserved for the present, the mind is often permanently enfeebled, and the patient ever afterwards unfitted for his ordinary vocations'. Some patients recovered to varying extents. The general belief held until comparatively recently that all serious illness required long bed rest would not have helped rehabilitation, and since most strokes are caused by blood clots in the brain, the immobility probably encouraged further clots. A small proportion of strokes are caused by a blood vessel rupturing in the brain – a 'cerebral haemorrhage'.

As far as treatments were concerned, most eighteenth and nineteenth-century doctors fell back on their core armamentarium for most ills – bloodletting, purges, vomiting, enemas, and blistering plasters. With ironic humour, poor Charles II apologised to his doctors after his stroke for spending so long dying whilst they tortured him with their useless but thoroughly unpleasant treatments. Many other patients must have suffered similar experiences.

Your Ancestors and Strokes

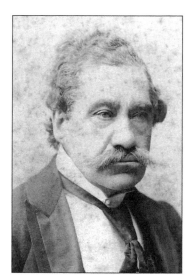

Gravestones and memorials sometimes indicate that an ancestor died very suddenly, and it's tempting to try and put a diagnosis to some of them. For example, a headstone in the churchyard of St Martin's Cathedral, Leicester reads: 'Beneath are deposited the remains of Richard Braginton – Quarter Master Sergeant of the South Devon

Subtle signs in this photograph of a Victorian ancestor suggest he may have suffered a stroke. The sitter's left lip pouts out, and his left lower eyelid is dragged down slightly compared to his right.

Militia – who expired suddenly in this town on his march to Nottingham in the night of the 15th of February 1812 after retiring to rest in perfect health. Aged 60 years.' A stroke would certainly be a contender as the cause of abrupt death without warning in an apparently healthy older man, but again a heart attack is another possibility. Many reported cases of apoplexy are in older persons, this report of an inquest in the *Salisbury and Winchester Journal*, 1825, being fairly typical: 'On Wednesday the 2nd inst. an inquest was taken by Mr Todd at Nether Wallop, on view of the body of Martha Cable, who, though advanced in years, enjoyed good health till Monday evening, when she was seized with apoplexy and soon after expired. Verdict – "Died by the Visitation of God".'

Occasionally you might find evidence for a stroke in a family photograph – maybe a lopsided appearance in the face or posture, or even a suggestion that, say, an arm is no longer fully functional.

Chapter 12

EXECUTION AND MURDER

Even though it might have happened hundreds of years ago, it can still be disturbing to find that one of your ancestors was deliberately killed. Murder takes many forms – an ancestor might be stabbed, shot, bludgeoned, strangled, drowned, starved, poisoned, crushed, or killed in any one of innumerable other cruel ways. The State, however, has traditionally chosen a more restricted range of methods for execution in the past few hundred years – principally hanging (sometimes with 'drawing and quartering'), beheading, and burning, although other methods were occasionally used. Military courts martial could lead to other forms of execution such as being shot by a firing squad or flogged to death.

Execution

The most notable trends in execution as a State punishment are that over the centuries it has gradually become less brutal, less public, and less frequently used. In Britain, the death sentence for murder was legally suspended in 1965 as an experiment, and then permanently abolished in 1969. The last hangings for murder were Peter Allen and Gwynne Evans in 1964. However, although not used after 1964, the death penalty stayed a legal option for certain crimes in Britain such as arson in a naval dockyard (until 1971), and spying (until 1981). The last two crimes that could legally attract the death penalty in Britain in peacetime were treason, and piracy with violence; capital punishment for these crimes was revoked only as recently as 1998.

Before the early nineteenth century, a large number of crimes still attracted the death penalty. Some of these seem shockingly trivial to us now, but earlier societies worked on the principle that execution was a valuable deterrent: killing a few individuals would prevent larger numbers of people breaking the law. What has become known as 'the bloody code' allowed execution for over 200 crimes, including attempted suicide, sheep stealing, homosexual sex, and theft from a church.

As an indication of the frequency of capital punishment, and the crimes for which it was most commonly invoked, the following table shows the numbers of executions carried out in London and Middlesex for the period 1756 to 1832:

Robbery	474
Burglary / house-breaking	454
Larceny	141
Murder	138
Forging currency ('coining')	76
Livestock stealing	53
Attempted murder	47
Forgery of wills etc.	30
Crimes against the post office	23
Rioting	20
Rape or paedophilia	18
Sodomy or bestiality	18
Arson	9
Smuggling	6
Sacrilege	1

It is interesting that executions for crimes against property (theft, forgery) predominate over those involving personal violence (murder, rape).

In practice, it was sometimes possible to work around the law's insistence on execution for certain less serious crimes. For example, a death sentence could be invoked but then rescinded after an appeal to a higher authority such as the monarch. Crimes against property were not liable to capital punishment if the value of the goods involved did not exceed a certain amount and so juries could deliberately undervalue what was stolen to avoid execution. However, by the beginning of the nineteenth century this was widely regarded as a deeply unsatisfactory state of affairs, and in 1823 Parliament passed the Judgement of Death Act, being 'an act for enabling courts to abstain from pronouncing death in certain capital felonies'.

One of the more gruesome aspects of State execution was the public exhibition of the victim's remains until they decayed 'as a warning to others'. This was known variously as gibbeting or 'hanging in chains', and it has taken various forms in the past but, remarkably, it continued to be legal in Britain until 1834.

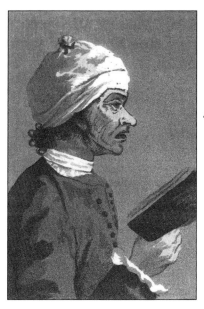

Theodore Gardelle, hanged in the Haymarket, London, in 1761 'amidst the shouts and hisses of an indignant populace' after which 'his body was hanged in chains upon Hounslow Heath'. He murdered Anne King, a woman of 'doubtful character' who was 'chiefly visited by gentlemen'.

Beheading

Traditionally a more noble or merciful form of death than others because it was quick, this form of execution was typically reserved for high-status victims and was used, for example, to dispatch Walter Raleigh, Anne Boleyn, Thomas Moore, and Mary Queen of Scots.

Burning

This barbaric practice has been a legal form of execution for crimes such as treason and heresy. In practice, most women convicted of witchcraft seem to have been hanged, although some were strangled first before burning. Notable executions include Janet Stewart and three other women who were tried for witchcraft in Edinburgh in 1597. They had been practising the art of healing using the traditional methods of the time but were also said to have employed 'charms'. They were condemned, taken to Castle Hill and there burned.

The definition of heresy and the frequency of executions for this crime vary considerably depending upon who was monarch. Notable persons burned for heresy include former Archbishop of Canterbury Thomas Cranmer, burned by order of Queen Mary I in 1556. The last person burned at the stake for heresy in England was the religious radical Edward Wightman who was executed at Lichfield in 1612.

It was not until the 1790s that burning ceased to be a legal method of execution, although long before it was abolished, those sentenced to death by this method were usually killed first. The last person burned by order of the State was a female forger, Christian Murphy, who was strangled then burned at the stake in 1789.

Hanging

This punishment was originally a slow death because the victim was allowed to dangle by a rope tied around the neck until he or she suffocated, which could take a surprisingly long time as the mid-Victorian *Medical Times and Gazette*, 1866, describes:

> Death is produced by hanging in one of three ways –
>
> Apoplexy; [a stroke]
> Asphyxia; [strangulation]
> Shock of the medulla oblongata caused by fracture of the vertebral column. [a 'broken neck']
>
> In the first two cases death is preceded by convulsions, lasting from five to forty-five minutes. In the third case death is instantaneous and painless, and this ought to be the aim of the hangman and the perfection of his art.

The highwayman Richard 'Dick' Turpin was hanged by this method on 7 April 1739 with a fellow offender, and the contemporary edition of the *Gentleman's Magazine* carried this account of his end:

> The notorious Richard Turpin, and John Stead, were executed at York for horse-stealing. Turpin behaved in an undaunted manner; as he mounted the ladder, feeling his right leg tremble, he stamp'd it down, and looking round about him with an unconcerned air, he spoke a few words to the topsman, then threw himself off, and expir'd in five minutes. He declared himself to be the notorious highwayman Turpin, and confess'd a great number of robberies, and that he shot the man that came to apprehend him on Epping Forest, and King his own companion, undesignedly, for which latter he was very sorry. He gave £3 10s to five men who were to follow the cart as mourners, with hatbands and gloves to them and several others. He was bury'd in St George's churchyard.

Unaccountably – by modern tastes – a public execution drew large crowds of onlookers who came to enjoy the spectacle. The governor of Devizes Prison recounted one such occasion in the *Mirror of Parliament*, 1841:

> The execution of James Moslin took place at this prison on the 6th September 1838, at 12 o'clock. By the time appointed for the execution, 15,000 persons must have congregated together. The most disgraceful and indecent behaviour pervaded the whole multitude. This exhibition must have operated very ineffectually upon the minds of a very large number of those who witnessed it; for in the after part of the day such scenes of drunkenness and debauchery have scarcely been witnessed. I may speak without compass when I say that not less than 2,000 persons, who came into the town to witness the scene, left in a state of beastly drunkenness. This number includes a very large portion of women, whose whole families accompanied them.

It was not until 1868 that public executions were banned, and from that date onwards all hangings were conducted behind prison walls.

The 'short drop' method of hanging, used in both the above cases, was replaced by a more humane approach in the late 1860s. The condemned individual fell through a trapdoor with the rope about the neck: when the rope pulled taut the victim's neck was broken so that death was almost instant. However, this method was made more precise by use of the 'long drop' method in the 1870s, with the length of the drop determined by the victim's body weight. Famous criminals who were hanged by this method include notorious murderer Charles Peace in 1879, Dr Hawley Harvey Crippen who poisoned his wife and was hanged in 1910, and Ruth Ellis, the last woman hanged in Britain in 1955.

Hanged, Drawn and Quartered

This gruesome death had a number of variants, but it generally involved being hanged until almost dead, and eviscerated whilst still alive. Then the body was chopped into four quarters, after removal of the head. From the eighteenth century onwards, executioners made sure the victim was hanged until dead, before cutting him open. The indignity of this form of execution meant that women were exempted from it and were generally burned or hanged instead.

Shortly after the Restoration of the monarchy, in 1660, the diarist Samuel Pepys attended the hanging drawing and quartering of Major

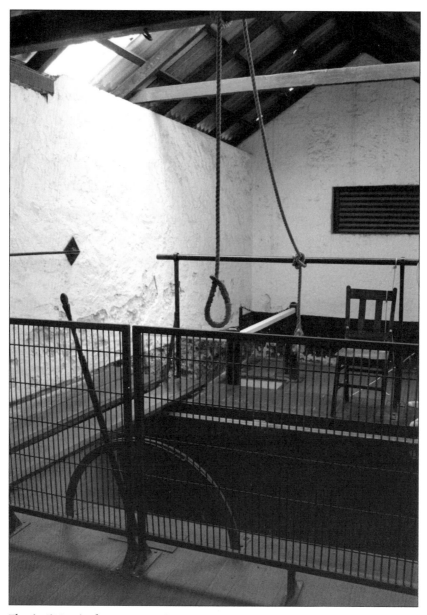

The facilities for hanging condemned prisoners at Fremantle prison, Australia, have been preserved and are the same as those that were used in Britain. The lever in the foreground has been pulled to the left to open the swing doors on which the victim would have stood with the noose around his neck.

General Thomas Harrison, who had been one of the signatories of Charles I's death warrant. The new king, Charles II, exacted a swift and brutal revenge for his father's execution, as Pepys recorded in his Diary: 'I went out to Charing Cross, to see Major-General Harrison hanged, drawn, and quartered; which was done there, he looking as cheerful as any man could do in that condition. He was presently cut down, and his head and heart shown to the people, at which there was great shouts of joy.'

In the seventeenth century, the words used by the judge to sentence a man to this form of death were quite explicit and not for the faint-hearted. For example, this was the sentence awarded upon the conviction of Lord William Russell for high treason in 1683:

> This court doth award that you be carried back again to the place from whence you came [i.e. prison], and from thence be drawn upon a hurdle to the place of execution where you shall be hanged up by the neck but cut down alive, your entrails and privy members [genitals] cut off from your body and burnt in your sight, your head to be severed from your body, and your body divided into four parts and disposed at the king's pleasure. And the Lord have mercy upon your soul.

Your Ancestors who were Executed or Murdered

Executions and investigations of murders involve legal proceedings, and so if you are researching an ancestor's fate in these circumstances your two principle sources of information will be criminal trial documents and newspaper reports of the case.

Legal Proceedings

Criminal records for England and Wales for 1791 to 1892 can be searched via the subscription website www.ancestry.co.uk .These are the digitised versions of TNA series HO 26 and HO 27, the earliest few years of which relate to Middlesex only. They describe trial outcomes and sentences, including executions. Proceedings from the Old Bailey for 1674 to 1913 are available free online at www.oldbaileyonline.org/, as are proceedings of the Court of Great Sessions in Wales 1730 to 1830 at www.llgc.org.uk/sesiwn_fawr/index_s.htm.

For example, in 1845, 21-year-old Emma Whiter was murdered in London. A search of the Old Bailey Online records or the criminal records on www.ancestry.co.uk using Emma's name or that of her alleged killer,

James Tapping, identifies the trial. The case was heard at the Old Bailey and the trial summary includes details of witness statements and questioning. Tapping was her lover and he was found guilty of shooting her in Bethnal Green with a pistol. He was sentenced to death.

Local archives tend to hold records of quarter sessions, local petty sessions and magistrates' courts. TNA's website has a research guide to British Army courts martial, www.nationalarchives.gov.uk, and also holds the records of the Justices of Assize from 1554 to 1971 in series ASSI, but these are not available online.

Coroners' inquiries into deaths are often kept in local archives or reported in newspapers, but TNA has a guide to finding the coroners' reports in its collection (see 'coroner' at www.nationalarchives.gov.uk/records/atoz).

Newspapers

Local and national newspapers are a good source of information about criminal trials. In the past – as is sometimes the case today – reporters had a tendency to become fixated on the more lurid aspects of the case and focus less on the details of the perpetrator's life and that of his or her victim. Chapter 2 gives details on how to access newspapers.

The case cited above, of the murder of Emma Whiter by James Tapping, attracted a lot of attention in the national newspapers of the time. Yet their focus was very much on the murderer and his remarkably cool demeanour and lack of remorse. Tapping became known as the 'Bethnal Green Murderer'. The *Illustrated London News*, for example, picked up the story on 1 February and ran with it for every edition until Tapping was hanged. This paper's detailed description of his execution on 29 March 1845 is instructive:

> EXECUTION OF THE BETHNAL GREEN MURDERER.
> On Monday morning, James Tapping was executed at Newgate, for the murder of Emma Whiter, at Bethnal Green.
> The conduct of the wretched man, both before and since conviction, was marked by the strictest propriety of demeanour.
> On Sunday he attended divine service in the prison chapel and passed the remainder of the day in the performance of his religious duties. The Rev. Mr. Davis was constantly in attendance upon him, but the day closed without any openly avowed expression of repentance. Tapping retired to rest about half-past ten o'clock that evening, and soon fell into a profound

sleep, from which he did not awake until half-past five o'clock on Monday morning. He then got up and dressed himself with more than ordinary attention to his toilet, remarking to one of the turnkeys, two of whom sat up with him every night since his conviction, 'That he did not know how it was, but he slept just as soundly in Newgate as he had been accustomed to do at home.'

On the morning of the execution, about seven o'clock, the culprit partook of breakfast, eating very heartily, and inviting the officers in attendance to do the same. Two cups of coffee, the same quantity of tea, two rolls, and a round of toast, formed the last meal of the wretched man.

At five minutes before eight o'clock, Calcraft, the executioner, was admitted to the cell for the purpose of performing the duties of his office. The awful symbols of the ignominious fate he was about to suffer, appeared not in the slightest degree to affect the prisoner. His firmness was perfectly astonishing.

Tapping bore the process of pinioning with the greatest fortitude, and so soon as it was completed, he turned to Mr. Sheriff Sydney, and said, 'I have one request to make, Sir; it is that I may be allowed to say a few words on the scaffold.'

The procession then moved forward, the rev. ordinary [Newgate's chaplain] reading the impressive service for the burial of the dead. On entering the prison from the chapel yard, the noise of the crowd congregated outside the walls re-echoed through the vaulted passages of the prison, but even this horrible harbinger of that which was to follow had no effect on the nerves of the prisoner. He walked erect, apparently the least moved of any person present, and really appeared to gain strength as he approached the fatal drop.

The wretched man mounted the scaffold without the slightest assistance, and walked deliberately forward towards the centre of the drop. In this position he stood for a moment, apparently contemplating the sea of upturned faces directed towards him. He then bowed thrice in a somewhat theatrical manner, turning himself successively to the west, north and south. This unusual movement was greeted by loud cheers and clapping of hands from the crowd. As soon as he had thus bowed, he appeared about to address the assemblage in front of the scaffold, but the buzz which arose from the mass of human beings congregated evidently convinced him that it was useless to attempt to make himself heard, and turning to the chaplain-and-ordinary, his last words were, 'I acknowledge the justice of my sentence, and I forgive everyone, as I hope by God's blessing to be forgiven.' He then shook hands successively with the executioner, the ordinary, and Mr. Sheriff Sydney, grasping the hands of the latter gentleman, and kissing them with great apparent fervour. The wretched man then resumed his position in the centre of the drop, and looked up with apparent curiosity at the beam and fatal chain. The cap was immediately drawn over his face, the rope adjusted, and the unfortunate felon, whose firm nerves never for a moment deserted him, was turned off, and died without a struggle.

Tapping was a young man of rather prepossessing appearance, and had scarcely completed his 22nd year. He wore a black velveteen shooting jacket and grey striped trousers, and had a very clean and neat appearance. The crowd at one period must have numbered between 6,000 and 7,000 persons. The majority seemed to have made their pilgrimage to Newgate the opening of a day's holiday.

Chapter 13

HEART CONDITIONS

Surprisingly, perhaps, heart conditions are not cited very frequently as a cause of death before the twentieth century. This is partly because our ancestors believed that the heart was not subject to disease and so cardiac disease went largely unrecognised before the nineteenth century, but also because serious heart conditions are generally a feature of older people, and in eras when many of our ancestors struggled to reach 50 years of age, then heart conditions appeared to be rare. When a 'heart attack' did occur it was often described as something else, e.g. 'apoplexy' (see below). It is also important to appreciate that the advent of certain types of heart diseases is influenced by lifestyle. Heart disease is much more common in modern times not only because people live longer but because heart disease is more likely in people who are overweight, eat a diet containing more fat, take little exercise, are stressed, and have a number of other risk factors which, by and large, affected our ancestors much less than they do people today.

Investigating Heart Disease

Over the centuries, doctors have slowly learned how the heart functions and how to assess it in disease. The first big milestone was the discovery by William Harvey in the early seventeenth century that the blood circulated around the body. The pulse had been used since ancient times to assess disease, but its real significance – that it was a sign of the heart pumping blood around the body – was not understood until Harvey's work. Nonetheless, measuring the speed of a patient's heartbeat by counting the pulse against a watch did not become routine practice until the nineteenth century.

Listening to a patient's chest is called auscultation. In antiquity, doctors put their ear directly to a person's bare chest to hear the heart. However, that great symbol of the doctor – the stethoscope – was developed by René Läennec in 1816. He used a wooden stick or tube with a cup at each

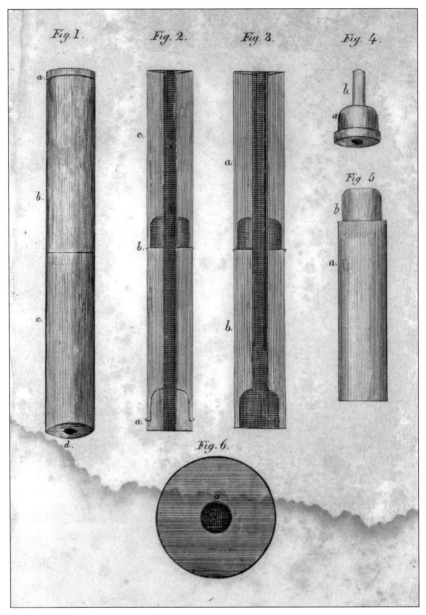

An early design of stethoscope from the 1820s.

end: one cup for the patient's chest and one for the doctor's ear. The more familiar modern form, using tubing that allows a doctor to listen with both ears, evolved in the mid-nineteenth century. This came into being at about the same time as the first blood-pressure monitoring apparatus (or sphygmograph), although the familiar variety used by doctors today with an inflatable cuff on the arm was not designed until the 1890s.

The electrocardiogram (ECG) machine was invented in the first years of the twentieth century. The earliest models weighed nearly 300kg and had to be operated by five people.

Heart Failure

Every pharmacist will tell you about William Withering. In the eighteenth century, his careful investigation and description of the medicinal properties of the foxglove plant, *Digitalis purpurea*, led to its being used as a heart medicine ever afterwards. And it is still prescribed today, although the isolated active ingredient, known as digoxin, is used rather than a plant extract.

Before it was recognised that the heart could grow weak and 'fail', doctors described these patients by their symptoms. Withering's foxglove extract was used to treat the condition known as dropsy – what we would now call water retention or oedema – a condition where fluid accumulates in the body making, for example, the ankles and belly swell. This is commonly caused by heart failure because the heart is not able to beat as powerfully as it once did. Sufferers also become short of breath, tired, and can tolerate little exercise. The term dropsy is a very old one, dating back to at least the thirteenth century, yet although we now often equate it with heart failure, a connection with the heart as a possible origin for the condition was not widely accepted until the nineteenth century.

Withering describes some cases in his published paper, *An Account of the Foxglove, and Some of Its Medical Uses*, 1785:

> Case 1. December 8th. A man about fifty years of age, who had formerly been a builder, but was now much reduced in his circumstances, complained to me of an asthma which first attacked him about the latter end of autumn. His breath was very short, his countenance was sunken, his belly large; and upon examination, a fluctuation in it was very perceptible. His urine for some time past had been small in quantity. I directed a decoction of Fol. Digital. recent. [digitalis extract] which made him very sick, the sickness recurring at intervals for several days, during which time he made a large quantity of water [urine]. His breath gradually drew easier, his belly subsided, and in about ten days he began to eat with a keen appetite.

Note that the term 'asthma' is here used as a general way to indicate a shortness of breath (see Chapter 6). Other terms to describe the breathing problems in heart failure included suffocative catarrh and dyspnoea. It should also be realised that not all cases of dropsy were caused by heart failure: fluid can build up in the body because of other medical conditions such as kidney disease. Foxglove only treats the heart-related causes.

But why did some people's hearts fail in the first place? This mystery that confronted doctors is eloquently summed up by the well-known nineteenth-century anatomist and surgeon George Murray Humphry in the *Provincial Medical and Surgical Journal*, 1850:

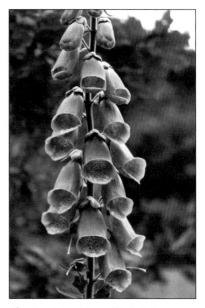

The foxglove plant (*digitalis*) was used successfully by William Withering to treat heart failure.

> In one man the heart goes on beating without fail through a long series of years, and at last ceases to contract, because the several organs are worn out, and fail to respond to one another and to supply the stimulus necessary for each other's action. In a second person, before half so many years have expired, the same organ, perhaps without giving any warning of its approaching failure, suddenly ceases to do its work, and its fibres are found to have lost their natural structure and to have transformed into oily matter. In a third person the valves, by repeated attacks of inflammation, become thickened, contracted and inefficient, so that the muscle labours on with difficulty, and at length is unable to overcome the obstacle so as to circulate blood enough to supply the wants of the system.

Most people's hearts lasted a lifetime, but some didn't. Some of those with failing hearts had damaged heart valves, as Humphry noted, and we now know that the repeated inflammation referred to by Humphry was often caused by infections such as rheumatic fever (see Chapter 7), which were much more common in the past.

Apart from digitalis, doctors used to bleed their patients, and in the nineteenth century, some doctors would open up some swollen areas of oedema to try and drain off the fluid. The first proper treatment to make patients urinate away some of the built-up fluid was mercury compounds given by injection in the 1930s; they forced patients' kidneys to pass more water, a job that by the 1960s could be done by taking 'water' tablets or diuretics.

The ultimate treatment for a weak or failing heart is to replace it, and Dr Christiaan Barnard performed the world's first human heart transplant operation in 1967.

Angina

Angina means 'strangling' in Greek and describes the pain in the chest that results from the heart not getting enough blood to feed itself with oxygen. It's like a heart attack (see below) that doesn't go the full distance. The pain usually goes away when sufferers sit down, try to relax, and get warm.

The first medical description of angina – or 'angina pectoris' to give it its full medical name – is usually credited to William Heberden in 1768, published in the *Medical Transactions of the College of Physicians* that year:

> They who are afflicted with it, are seized while they are walking (more especially if it be uphill, and soon after eating), with a painful and most disagreeable sensation in the breast, which seems as if it would extinguish life if it were to increase or continue; but the moment they stand still, all this uneasiness vanishes.
>
> In all other respects, the patients are, at the beginning of the disorder, perfectly well and in particular have no shortness of breath, from which it is totally different. The pain is sometimes situated in the upper part, sometimes in the middle, sometimes at the bottom of the *os sterni* [breastbone], and often more inclined to the left than to the right side. It likewise very frequently extends from the breast to the middle of the left arm. Males are most liable to that disease, especially such as have passed their fiftieth year.

Heberden goes on to say that he has little advice on treatment, except quiet and warmth after an attack, but that this lack of knowledge would be expected since angina has 'hitherto hardly had a place or a name in medical books'. However, he adds 'I knew one who set himself a task of sawing wood for half an hour every day, and was nearly cured'. If you ask any modern-day angina sufferer if they would like to saw up wood every day you may not receive a polite answer – it is an exercise very likely to bring on angina pain, not cure it.

One of the first successful treatments for angina was literally explosive. Nitroglycerine (or glyceryl trinitrate) is used to make dynamite. People in the Victorian factories that made or packed it, used to get a headache on Monday mornings, and it was also noticed that workers with a history of angina would suffer at weekends, but not during the working week when they were handling the explosive. Both these effects were caused by nitroglycerine opening up the workers' blood vessels – in the head this caused a headache; near the heart it relieved the pressure on a strained system and stopped the angina pain. This treatment is still used today to relieve an angina attack, with most patients now carrying a glyceryl trinitrate or 'GTN' spray around with them in case they need it.

Heart Attacks

A heart attack is also known as a coronary thrombosis (a 'coronary') or myocardial infarction. It is also one of the likely causes of the 'sudden death' sometimes cited on death certificates, and of 'apoplexy' which, although traditionally referring to a stroke, was actually applied to any sudden collapse and death (see Chapter 11).

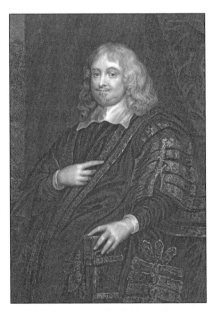

The usual cause of a heart attack is a blood clot in one of the blood vessels that gives the heart its own blood supply (a coronary artery). As a result, the heart cannot get enough of the oxygen and nutrients that normally fuels its activity. This causes a crushing or pressing pain in the centre of the chest that often radiates into the arms and throat, and the affected person usually collapses.

Edward Hyde, Earl of Clarendon died of a heart attack in 1674 at a time when doctors did not believe the heart was subject to disease.

As noted in the introduction to this chapter, heart disease tends to affect older persons and so accounts of it before the nineteenth century are not common. Some probable accounts of a heart attack seem to have perplexed the physicians of the time who were not used to seeing it. For example, the death of Edward Hyde, Earl of Clarendon, in 1674 bears all the signs of a heart attack, as is evidenced by this extract from *The Life of Edward, Earl of Clarendon*:

[He] went to the church to a sermon, where he found himself a little pressed [chest pain, i.e. angina] as he used to be, and therefore thought fit to make what haste he could to his house, and was no sooner come thither into a lower room, than having made water [urinated], and the pain in his arm seizing upon him, he fell down dead without the least motion of any limb: the suddenness of it made it apprehended to be apoplexy [a stroke], but there being nothing like convulsions, or the least distortion or alteration in the visage, it is not like to be from that cause; nor could the physicians make any reasonable guess from whence that mortal blow proceeded. He wanted about six weeks of attaining the age of seventy. [1827 edition.]

Even in the late nineteenth century, doctors were still confused about the difference between angina and heart attacks. Hence an ancestor noted as dying of 'angina' would probably have suffered what we would now call a heart attack. It was not until the 1930s that the diagnosis of a heart attack acquired a surer footing, and then mainly because it was becoming a lot more common and therefore more familiar and easier to study.

As the twentieth century progressed, the frequency of heart attacks increased with every decade, as life expectancy rose together with the heart-unfriendly behaviours already alluded to at the beginning of this chapter (poor diet etc.). Heart attacks could only be managed by treating the sufferer's symptoms, using whatever medicines or techniques were available at the time – none of which were particularly effective. Until the 1980s the chances of dying from a heart attack in Britain stood at about 1 in 4, with more dying in the aftermath.

More recently preventative medicines, health education, and clot-busting drugs have dramatically reduced the risks of dying from a heart attack.

Chapter 14

INFLUENZA

Influenza or 'flu' is caused by a virus, and in recent centuries has proved liable periodically to spread worldwide in the form of a pandemic. In the past it has also been called the grippe (especially in North America and Continental Europe), epidemic catarrh, catarrhal fever, and feveret.

The term *influenza* was first used in English in the eighteenth century and is the Italian word for 'influence' – perhaps originally because it was believed that the progress of this and other contagious diseases was under the influence of the stars. The word was first associated with a particularly virulent European epidemic which was believed to have spread to Britain from Italy in 1743.

The influenza virus mutates to form different strains and these can affect how quickly the disease spreads and the symptoms it causes. So, for example, the seasonal flu that occurs in the winter each year has different characteristics to the pandemic form of the disease which is not seasonal, spreads around the globe, and can occur at any time of the year. Pandemic flu is also more virulent and more likely to kill the sufferer.

Symptoms
The symptoms of flu can be rather non-specific, which may make it difficult sometimes to determine if historical accounts do refer to the disease. Symptoms can also vary quite a lot according to the individual and the strain of influenza virus. Yet influenza is characterised by an ability to spread and infect a large number of people quickly. The classic features are: fever, headache, aching muscles and joints, a runny nose, sore throat, and a cough. Usually these last for five days or so, but they can persist for longer and may predispose the weakened sufferer to chest infections such as pneumonia.

The very young and the very old are most likely to be killed by seasonal flu, although in a pandemic – when as many as 1 per cent of sufferers may die – people are liable to die at any age, including young and fit adults. Those who have survived any form of flu often feel lethargic and withdrawn for some time afterwards.

Historical Epidemics

In Britain, influenza epidemics have occurred several times each century since the mid-1500s, and some were more lethal than others. The outbreak of influenza in Elizabethan England in 1558 may have killed about 5 per cent of the population, and the peak months for deaths were August and September.

The physician Thomas Sydenham describes a seventeenth-century epidemic, reproduced in John Pechey's *The Whole Works of that Excellent Practical Physician Dr Thomas Sydenham*, 1734:

> When a pleasant and warm season like summer held to the end of October – contrary to custom – in the year 1675, a cold and moist season came presently after, and there were more coughs than ever I knew at any other time, sparing scarce anybody of whatever age or temperament, and seizing whole families together. Nor were they remarkable only for their number, for every winter there are many, but also upon account of the danger which they cast those into accidentally that had them. For the constitution being now, and all the foregoing autumn, very inclinable to produce the epidemic fever … these coughs made way for the fever, and easily turned into it … For now as always before, it began with a pain in the head, the back, and limbs.
>
> In November in the foresaid year, Mr Thomas Windham, the eldest son of Sir Francis Windham, was my patient; in this fever he complained of a pain in the side and other symptoms wherewith others were afflicted that had this disease. I bled him once, and applied a blister to his neck; clysters [enemas] were daily injected, and he drank cooling ptisans [medicinal drinks] and emulsions, and sometimes milk-water or small beer, and I advised that he should keep from bed for some hours. And by this method he recovered within a few days, and purging [laxatives] being used, he was quite well.

Part of Sydenham's treatment of his case actually mirrors twenty-first-century practice quite well: plenty of fluids to drink, and rest. It's a shame about the gratuitous bleeding, blistering, and enemas.

There were several influenza epidemics in the eighteenth and nineteenth centuries. The peak years for influenza do vary somewhat according to the sources used, but I have relied upon those identified by Theophilus Thompson in his book *Annals of Influenza or Epidemic Catarrhal Fever in Great Britain 1510 to 1837*. He identifies the following years as periods of intense influenza activity in Britain after 1650 by relying on contemporary accounts of disease activity: 1658, 1675, 1688, 1693, 1709, 1729, 1737, 1743, 1758, 1762, 1767, 1775, 1782, 1789–90, 1803, 1831, and 1833. There were later pandemics that affected Britain in 1836, 1843, 1848, 1855, 1870, and 1889–92, the last of these being the so-called 'Russian flu'.

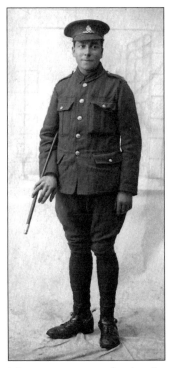

Many young men who fought in the First World War and survived it died of Spanish flu in the aftermath.

The cruellest, and certainly the most overwhelming, influenza pandemic was that which began during the final phase of the First World War in 1918. Known as 'Spanish flu', it killed at least 50 million people worldwide at a time when many populations were overcome and demoralised by the effects of war. That war had killed greater numbers of people than any other conflict known at the time, but the flu killed far more: it is the single most lethal influenza pandemic known in history.

The relocation and demobilisation of large numbers of troops after the war may have helped to ensure the rapid spread of Spanish flu, but the strain of virus itself seems to have been particularly virulent. It caused the deaths mainly of young adults, and produced a much higher mortality rate than other pandemics, with around 10 per cent or more of those infected dying. This was devastating for families and societies after the loss of so many young people in five years of global conflict. The pandemic eventually dissipated by the end of 1920.

There were two other pandemics in the twentieth century – in 1957 ('Asian flu') and 1968 ('Hong Kong flu'), but these were much less deadly.

Influenza vaccines were first developed in the 1940s, but have only been recommended in Britain since the late 1960s.

Chapter 15

MENTAL ILLNESS AND SUICIDE

Psychiatric conditions have often been poorly understood, so men and women with mental illness were sometimes treated very cruelly in the past. Our distant ancestors believed the moon affected human behaviour, and the word 'lunatic' comes from the Latin word for moon, *luna*. Lunatics were sometimes sane and sometimes not – waxing and waning like the moon.

Many of our ancestors considered mental illness shameful and embarrassing, and people who suffered from it were often regarded as weak, stupid, or degenerate. Sufferers receiving medical attention were often 'put away' in asylums or similar institutions and then no longer discussed in public.

Asylums

Asylums were places of refuge, and so finding an ancestor in an asylum may not indicate mental illness. There were asylums for the blind, retired seamen, orphans, and so forth.

However, lunatic asylums, or madhouses, arose because lunatics were feared and because they couldn't necessarily fend for themselves. Asylums enabled them to be shut away where they could be controlled. There were two kinds of lunatic asylum. Private asylums were run for those who could pay for a relative to be detained, whereas county asylums served the wider community. There were few county asylums before the nineteenth century, but they increased in number following an Act of Parliament in 1808, and again in 1845 when it became compulsory for counties to provide them.

Asylums were subject to great abuse, especially before 1850, and most were simply places of confinement. Conditions were often harsh: inmates could be chained or tied up if they didn't obey the staff, and there was little exercise, entertainment, or anything like what we would call 'treatment'. Unscrupulous individuals could pay corrupt asylum officials to have people 'locked away' without too many questions being asked. The following extract is taken from the *Gentleman's and London Magazine*, 1763:

> A bill of indictment was found by the grand jury of Westminster against the master and servants of a certain mad house, for unjustly detaining a young gentleman 13 months, and using him cruelly. It is said his pretended friends met him on board an Indiaman [a ship], and took him with his effects – which were considerable – into a coach and, instead of taking him home as they pretended, carried him to this mad house where, though in his perfect senses, he was confined in a strait waistcoat, tied down 17 nights and days, denied the use of pen, ink, and paper, and otherwise used so ill that he spit blood. But at length, by getting some Morella cherries and a toothpick, he found means to let his case be known to an acquaintance, who soon after procured his liberty.

The use of cherries and toothpicks to escape illegal confinement is most intriguing!

Before the county asylums came into being, poor people with mental illness – or 'pauper lunatics' – that were not cared for by their families were often put in workhouses, or even prison. There was no organised system of care for them.

Britain's first and most famous asylum was the Hospital of St Mary Bethlem, known as 'Bedlam', and now as Bethlem Royal Hospital in London. It originated in the sixteenth century, and the conditions for inmates were wretched – cramped and foul-smelling, and filled with noisy and distressed people. The public were allowed to pay a penny to see and taunt the patients. This shameful pursuit was so popular that it brought the hospital the princely income of £400 per year in 1770. As late as 1814, the patients' small squalid rooms were described as 'dog kennels' with many people chained to the wall.

Yet in common with many other asylums, conditions did slowly improve. In 1843, a reporter from the *Illustrated London News* remarked that,

> the scrupulous cleanliness of the house, the decent attire of the patients, and the unexpectedly small number of those under restraint ... lead the visitor to conclude that the management of lunatics has here attained perfection; whilst the quiet and decent

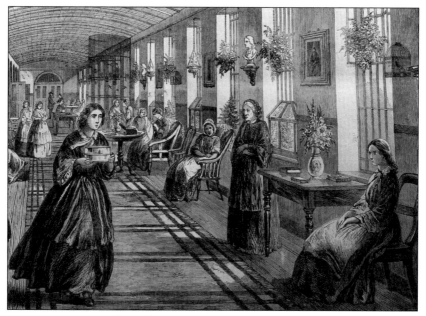

Female inpatients at the Bethlem Royal Hospital in 1860.

demeanour of the inmates might almost make him doubt that
he is really in a madhouse.

Although asylum security was effective when it came to preventing the
patients escaping, it failed to protect them from abuse by other patients
and even staff. This applied to both private asylums and their county
equivalents. The following disturbing extract is taken from the *Lancet*,
January 1868:

A female inmate of the Abergavenny Lunatic Asylum was
recently found dead in her bed, with an apron-string tightly
around her neck; and on post-mortem examination it was
discovered that, in addition to the strangulation, which was the
immediate cause of death, the deceased bore on her chest deep
marks of the knuckles of a person's hand, and that one of her
ribs was broken. Medical evidence showed that none of the
injuries could have been self-inflicted, and at the inquest it was
stated that the apron to which the string belonged was
sufficiently peculiar to be identified as one which on the
morning of the death had been given to another inmate who
was, however, in so excited a condition as to be unable to give

any intelligible or reliable evidence. It appears that the deceased had been for some time confined to her bed, and that she had been visited by the nurse only two hours before the time that she was found dead. The finding of the coroner's jury was that 'the deceased was strangled by some person unknown'; but inferentially, it seems probable that the murder was committed by the inmate in possession of the apron. What sort of supervision is that which admits of one inmate going to the bedside of another and, after inflicting injuries which must have caused some outcry on the part of the victim, carrying out the leisurely process of strangulation?

Asylum Staff

In the eighteenth and nineteenth centuries, asylums employed 'lunatic keepers' to supervise patients. In smaller asylums the owner was often the head keeper; in larger establishments keepers were drawn from all walks of life but typically from labouring classes. They were frequently men who were physically imposing and strong so that they could overawe and restrain the patients. The pay was not good, but did include onsite lodging and food. Sometimes keepers had to stay single to keep their position, but in smaller asylums the keeper's wife and family might work with him in varying capacities – preparing food, washing clothes, cleaning, and so forth.

Staffing levels were low, but keepers were often helped to manage their patients by other staff known as attendants or assistants, and there were usually female employees to look after the women. Asylum workers gained their experience on the job, and no previous experience was generally deemed necessary. Some were even ex-patients.

Until the mid-nineteenth century, the prevailing approach to lunatics was that they were at best unpredictable, at worst dangerous. Consequently, the keeper's primary

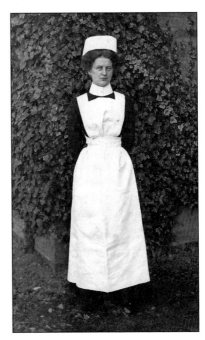

Ruth Coates, a nurse at Warwick County Lunatic Asylum, Hatton, in 1905.

role was to control patients by virtually any means possible. This could include forced restraint, violence, and various other punishments such as immersion in cold water.

County asylums generally employed doctors, but many private asylums did not until later Victorian times. In the second half of the nineteenth century, asylums began to employ nurses and matrons.

Causes and Treatments

In 1758, William Battie published his *Treatise on Madness*. He advocated asylums as places where patients should avoid things that upset them. In a swipe at Bethlem, Battie pleaded that 'the impertinent curiosity of those that think it pastime to converse with madmen and to play upon their passions ought strictly to be forbidden'. He proposed that madness be managed by identifying and treating its causes, then attending to specific symptoms.

He classified madness into two kinds: 'original madness' was natural to the person, whereas 'consequential madness' had a definite cause (e.g. a head injury). However, his list of causes was very much a product of the times and included 'tumultuous passions' such as joy and anger, exposure to the sun, gluttony, alcohol, idleness, and 'unwearied attention of the mind to one object, or from the quieter passions of love, grief, and despair'.

Battie concluded that whilst consequential madness was treatable, 'original madness is not curable by any method which human reason or experience hath hitherto been able to discover'. This was the general conclusion of most authorities until the twentieth century, so patients were put away where they could be managed behind closed doors.

Treatment slowly began to become more humane in the nineteenth century thanks largely to the example set by certain Christian organisations, including the Quakers.

Electricity began to be used to treat some forms of severe mental illness in the late 1930s, and this electroconvulsive therapy or 'ECT' is still used. However, a number of radical treatments were employed around this time that are no longer used including surgery on the brain, such as a 'lobotomy'. Various medicines were tried over the centuries to treat mental illness, but with little good effect: in Victorian times, some doctors used opium because its sedative action was believed to calm the patient. Chlorpromazine was the breakthrough prescription medicine for schizophrenia-type disorders ('psychoses') in the 1950s, and the first effective antidepressants for general use also became available in this decade.

Suicide

An ancestor taking his or her own life is a particularly tragic event to uncover when researching your family's history. Not all suicides are the result of mental illness: suicide as a reaction to personal tragedy could be considered a noble act or even an obligation in ancient times. For example, the Roman senator Cato chose to take his life when his forces were about to be defeated by Julius Caesar. In more recent centuries there are many instances of someone committing suicide for identifiable reasons: because of financial ruin, disgrace, unrequited love, or physical illness, for example. These all illustrate that suicide can be a voluntary, pre-meditated act as a reaction to events.

Yet it is well established that a serious psychiatric disorder does increase the risk of suicide. In particular, the prolonged sadness and feelings of helplessness caused by depression is strongly linked to an increased risk, as this account, published in the *Devizes and Wiltshire Gazette*, 4 July 1839, illustrates:

> On Sunday last, Mrs. Brown, of Harnham, went as usual to attend divine service, leaving her sister, Mrs. Mary Morris, at home in bed, suffering from severe indisposition; but on her return she was horror-struck on finding that the poor woman had quitted her own apartment, and, on searching for her, she discovered her corpse suspended by a silk-handkerchief from the upper rail of a small bedstead, in one of the attics. Life was quite extinct, and there can be no doubt that the unfortunate creature had perpetrated the awful act soon after she was left alone. An inquest was held on Monday evening, before R.M. Wilson, esq., Coroner for Salisbury, when it appeared from the evidence, that the deceased, who was in her 66th year, had formerly been in prosperous if not in affluent circumstances; but of late years had been afflicted by several apoplectic seizures, which had destroyed her health, and irretrievably depressed her spirits. It was also proved that she suffered from occasional aberrations of mind; and a respectable jury, after patiently investigating all the facts returned a verdict of lunacy.

The means of killing oneself have changed a little with the era. Since Victorian times, the commonest methods have been hanging, drowning, poisoning (including overdose), and cutting oneself to bleed to death. However, when domestic gas supplies came into widespread use in around 1920 there was a very marked increase in the use of this method for suicide, and gassing became the single most popular technique used by both sexes from the late 1920s to about 1970. In the 1860s, poisoning accounted for about 5 per cent of suicides, with acids being the commonest agents (e.g. hydrochloric, carbolic, and oxalic acids); by the 1990s self-poisoning represented about 22 per cent of suicides with medicines such as painkillers and antidepressants being the most common means.

Data from 1860 to the 1980s generally show an increased risk of suicide with age: those over 55 years of age being at highest risk. The highest rates of suicide ever recorded were in the aftermath of the Great Depression in the 1930s: the peak year was 1934 with over 4 in every 10,000 deaths in England and Wales recorded as a suicide. This is about three times the incidence seen in the early twenty-first century. There was also a peak in around 1905 and in the 1960s.

There are some differences between the sexes. The incidence of suicide in men has always been higher than in women, and men are also more likely to be successful when suicide is attempted. Between 1860 and 2000, between one-and-a-half and four times more men than women committed suicide in England and Wales in any given year. Men are more likely to adopt violent means of suicide than women, and so there is a greater incidence of hanging, jumping to one's death, and use of firearms amongst males.

Suicide posed many legal and religious problems for our ancestors. It is somewhat ironic that suicide was illegal in Britain until 1961. The eighteenth-century legal thinking behind this approach was explained by a former Solicitor General, William Blackstone, in *Commentaries on the Laws of England*, 1765:

> The law of England wisely and religiously considers that no man hath a power to destroy life but by commission from God, the author of it: and as the suicide is guilty of a double offence – one spiritual in invading the prerogative of the Almighty and rushing into his presence uncalled for, the other temporal against the King who hath an interest in the preservation of all his subjects – the law has therefore ranked this among the highest crimes, making it a peculiar species of felony: a felony committed on oneself.
>
> … But now the question follows, what punishment can human laws inflict on one who has withdrawn himself from their reach? They can only act upon what he has left behind him, his reputation and fortune: on the former, by an

> ignominious burial in the highway, with a stake driven through his body; on the latter, by a forfeiture of all his goods and chattels to the king: hoping that his care for either his own reputation, or the welfare of his family, would be some motive to restrain him from so desperate and wicked an act.

Despite the disapproval of God and the monarch, and the risk of having one's family disinherited after death, suicides still happened. For one thing, what the law said and what actually happened in practice were often different. Communities might enforce the strict letter of the law about property, and the local church might refuse an orthodox burial, but this didn't always happen and attitudes to suicide softened with time.

The burial of suicide victims in particular was the subject of special legal and religious consideration in the past – not all were buried at a highway with a stake through the body as Blackstone advised above, although it was widely practised, and as late as the early nineteenth century. This rather heartless custom was not officially halted until the Burial of Suicide Act in 1823, which mandated that suicides be interred in the parish burial ground privately – i.e. without any of the usual rites of Christian burial. Society's disapproval of suicide meant that this burial had to take place in darkness between the hours of 9 o'clock and midnight. The church might refuse to inter the body on consecrated ground, but churchyards and public cemeteries generally had a section of unconsecrated ground set aside for this and other purposes. In 1882, a further Act allowed the body of a suicide victim to be interred with full religious ceremony in the same way as any other corpse. However, the burial of a person committing suicide might often not be recorded in the parish register before this date.

Your Ancestors and Mental Illness

There is more scope to research ancestors with mental illness than probably any other health topic, and a range of information resources are available.

Censuses

The census may allow you to identify ancestors resident in asylums. Unfortunately, some individuals were only identified by their initials to provide confidentiality. From 1871, there was a column in the census return to indicate whether someone was a lunatic, imbecile, or idiot. From 1901, 'idiot' was replaced with 'feeble-minded'.

Lunatics tended to be people suffering from schizophrenia-like illnesses, whereas an 'idiot' was born with mental incapacity. An 'imbecile' was someone whose mental state deteriorated during adulthood so that they became 'infantile'.

Local Records

Asylums were distributed all around the country, so there is no centralised index to inpatients. Most records are kept by the regional archive in the county where the asylum was based. You can find their location by searching the website of the archive concerned, and TNA's HospRec database at www.nationalarchives.gov.uk/hospitalrecords/. If your searches here are unsuccessful try the National Register of Archives at www.nationalarchives.gov.uk/nra and Access to Archives at www.nationalarchives.gov.uk/a2a.

If you do not have a complete name for the asylum, or do not know where it was located, then Middlesex University's asylum index will help you at http://studymore.org.uk/4_13_ta.htm. Some asylums changed their names, and records may only be indexed under the most recent name.

Twentieth-century records may be subject to varying degrees of non-disclosure, depending on whether individuals can be identified or not. Archivists will be able to tell you what you can and can't look at.

The most consistently preserved records are admissions books. They vary quite a lot in the detail they provide, but commonly give the

The Royal Albert Asylum for Idiots in Lancaster, which was intended 'for the care, education and training of feeble-minded children and young persons'.

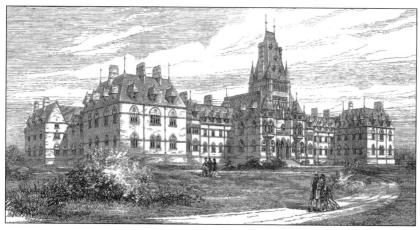

patient's name, age, diagnosis, address, and next of kin. They often reveal that, despite the popular perception, many patients were admitted for a short time and then discharged. For example, the admissions book for Hampshire County Lunatic Asylum shows that on 25 March 1856 William Taylor, a 27-year-old miller, was admitted suffering from mania. He lived in Carisbrooke on the Isle of Wight and his brother, James, an accountant from Fareham agreed to pay for his keep. His illness had begun the year before and was attributed to 'being frightened as a child'. He was noted to be 'in enfeebled bodily health and condition', but was discharged as recovered two months later.

Other asylum records can include discharge registers, administrative papers that sometimes mention individual patients, and very occasionally doctors' more detailed accounts of individuals and their treatments.

A few records have been digitised and are available online. Prestwich Asylum records, for example, are available to view at www.findmaypast. co.uk (subscription required).

TNA Records

The Lunacy Commission (later the Board of Control) kept inpatient registers for county asylums between 1846 and 1960. This is series MH 94 and it lists patient names by date of admission only – there is no name index – but it does identify the asylum, and dates of discharge or death. The registers are split into various categories such as voluntary admissions, paupers etc., so you may need to look through several if you don't know the precise details. Private asylums are not included, but a register of admissions to certain private asylums outside London is kept as series MH 51/735 covering 1798–1812; it also identifies keepers.

Certain parts of series MH at TNA can contain detailed descriptions of individual patients' cases – for example, series MH 85, MH 86 and MH 51/27-77. You can hunt through these by patient name to see if your ancestor's treatment details are referenced using the 'search within' function in the advanced search of TNA's discovery service at http://discovery.nationalarchives.gov.uk.

Specialist asylums took patients from a much wider geographical area and include those for the criminally insane or ex-servicemen. For example, TNA keeps records for lunatic navy personnel admitted to Hoxton House (1755–1818) and Haslar (1818–54) as series ADM 102/415-20 and ADM 102/356-73. Criminal lunatics are identified in a variety of records at TNA including HO 8 (1862–76) and HO 145 (1882–1921). There is a one-off listing of all insane prisoners for 1858 arranged by prison in series MH 51/90-207.

Apart from criminality, there were many situations in which a person's mental health might be a legal issue. Were they fit to manage their estate? Or to make a will? Series C 211 at TNA are records of commissions and inquisitions to determine lunacy (1627–1932). They are indexed by name in TNA's Catalogue: input an ancestor's surname and restrict to series C 211. Do not use complete names as some are indexed in the form 'Charles Clarke', others as 'Clarke, Charles'.

Workhouses

Pauper lunatics were commonly accommodated in workhouses, and there may be local records of this. However, details of workhouse inmates are also kept at TNA in series MH 12 (1833–1909), although most content is not concerned with mental illness. Some records have been digitised, and can be searched via TNA's Discovery service by name of individual or Poor Law union. If visiting TNA to search MH 12, note that it is

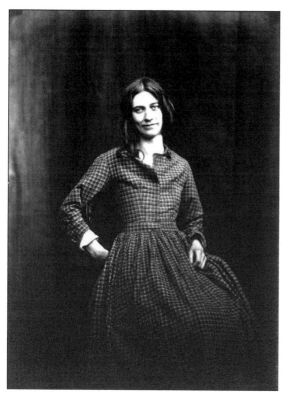

This inpatient in Surrey County Lunatic Asylum was photographed in the 1850s.

indexed first by county and then by name of Poor Law union. For example, MH 12/690 is part of the Cambridgeshire series, but specifically for Newmarket 1854–5.

Mental Health Terminology

Mental illness was often described by generalised or poorly defined terms in former times such as 'of unsound mind'. Similarly, the word 'dementia' means 'without a mind' and was used to describe a range of conditions. Some other examples of terminology are given below:

- Cretin – mental illness in an infant caused by thyroid disease.
- Exhaustion (of the vital powers) – probably depression.
- Hysteria, 'the vapours' – an over-emotional or excitable state usually applied to women. Probably would be called a panic attack or an anxiety disorder today.
- Lunacy, insanity, madness, or derangement of the mind – although fairly imprecise, they often applied to schizophrenia or psychosis.
- Mania – bipolar disorder.
- Melancholia, despondency – depression.
- Natural decay, senility, imbecile, old-age decline, feeble-minded – often referred to old-age dementia.
- Nerves, nerve trouble – anxiety.
- Paralysis, palsy, effusion on the brain – often a stroke.
- Mongolism – Down's syndrome.
- Shell shock – post-traumatic stress disorder.

Chapter 16

OPIUM ADDICTION

Addiction is not simply a modern phenomenon. Indeed, there are three substances with a comparatively long history of human addiction that are still with us today in one form or another: alcohol (see Chapter 4), tobacco (Chapter 6), and finally opium from which drugs such as heroin were later derived. The abuse of other substances to the point where addiction occurs – such as cocaine and amphetamines – is a relatively recent development in Britain that started in the twentieth century.

The Opium Flower

The story of opium is rather like the story of Dr Jekyll and Mr Hyde. On the one hand opium is a plant that has enabled freedom from suffering, wealth, and happiness; but on the other hand it has brought despair, war, and death.

The opium poppy is native to southern Europe and western Asia, and has been used by humans as a medicine and intoxicant for at least 6,000 years. Its Latin name is *Papaver somniferum*, which means the poppy that brings sleep, reflecting the long-attested use of the plant as a sedative. The opium poppy is the only species that has this property – the common red field poppies of Britain, for example, do not produce these effects.

The opium flower has a central capsule which swells once the petals start to be lost. In nature, this capsule holds the seeds of future generations, but when raised as a crop the capsule is slit before it matures and the oozing sap is harvested as a congealed 'latex'. This is opium, which contains morphine as its most important constituent.

A surprising source for a description of raw opium, perhaps, is Mrs Beeton. Opium was the only reliable painkiller available to the Victorians so it was widely used. In her *Book of Household Management* (1861), Isabella Beeton (1836–65) advises several uses for the drug. She says: 'Solid opium is mostly seen in the form of rich brown flattish cakes, with

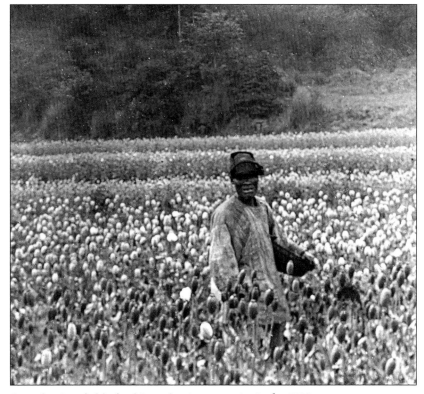

A worker in a field of cultivated opium poppies in the 1880s.

little pieces of leaves sticking on them here and there, and a bitter and slightly warm taste.' Members of the public could buy raw opium, or get it ready made into various medicines.

Opium Medicines

The seventeenth-century physician Thomas Sydenham asserted the value of opium with great enthusiasm:

> The wonderful effects of opium are owing to the native goodness and excellency of the plant that affords it … Moreover, this medicine is so necessary an instrument in the hands of a skilful person, that the art of physic would be defective and imperfect without it; and whoever is thoroughly acquainted with its virtues, and the manner of using it will perform greater things than might reasonably be expected from the use of any single medicine. [Reproduced in *The Entire Works of Dr Thomas Sydenham*, ed. John Swan, 1742 edn.]

The drug allowed people to recover painlessly from traumatic injuries and from surgery, it was calming, alleviated cough, stopped diarrhoea, and it helped sleep. Opium's effects were so remarkable that they could only be a divine gift. Even today, the Royal College of Anaesthetists acknowledges the importance of opium to medical history by including the flower in its coat of arms.

The effects of opium had been well known in Britain for centuries, but it was not until the seventeenth century that its use became more widespread. This happened because in Turkey and Asia opium began to be grown on a large scale as a commercial crop, and the expansion of trade allowed the drug to be imported in bigger quantities. At this time, opium's main use was medicinal, yet as early as 1704 one authority wrote: 'It would be endless to give all the preparations we meet with of this most celebrated drug.' Everyone had their favourite formula, and because sales were unrestricted by law, anyone could buy or sell opium. Nonetheless, the three most familiar forms were:

- Laudanum (also known as tincture of opium) consisted of opium dissolved in alcohol.
- Paregoric (camphorated tincture of opium) was opium in alcohol, with camphor and other pleasant-smelling ingredients.
- Opium pills of varying formulas.

However, as the eighteenth century advanced the public was confronted with a growing number of brand-name products containing opium, often called patent medicines. Many of these even had secret formulas. Opium is a very potent medicine and it was used to treat a wide range of inappropriate medical conditions including teething troubles and colic in infants, anxiety, food poisoning, mental illness, and tuberculosis. It is easy to be critical of this laissez-faire approach, but at the time there were no other painkillers – no paracetamol or aspirin – and few medicines that effectively treated common ailments such as diarrhoea or insomnia. Yet opium was a gift from nature, and it was not considered harmful.

Addiction

In 1821, Thomas de Quincey published a landmark book, *Confessions of an English Opium Eater*. As the title suggests, it was one man's personal account of his experiments with taking opium and his eventual dependency. It was a revelation and a best-seller in Victorian times because no one had ever written anything like this before. De Quincey took opium originally to cure a headache, but became a long-term user.

After his first dose he declared: 'Here was a panacea for all human woes; here was the secret of happiness, about which philosophers had disputed for so many ages, at once discovered; happiness might now be brought for a penny, and carried in the waistcoat-pocket'. The book still offers a fascinating insight into one man's experiences and can be read online at www.gutenberg.org/etext/2040, although the style is often over-sentimental and rambling. De Quincey is keen to show the widespread nature of addiction:

> Three respectable London druggists, in widely remote quarters of London, from whom I happened lately to be purchasing small quantities of opium, assured me that the number of amateur opium-eaters (as I may term them) was at this time immense; and that the difficulty of distinguishing those persons to whom habit had rendered opium necessary from such as were purchasing it with a view to suicide, occasioned them daily trouble and disputes. This evidence respected London only. But – which will possibly surprise the reader more – some years ago, on passing through Manchester, I was informed by several cotton manufacturers that their workpeople were rapidly getting into the practice of opium-eating; so much so, that on a Saturday afternoon the counters of the druggists were strewed with pills of one, two, or three grains, in preparation for the known demand of the evening. The immediate occasion of this practice was the lowness of wages, which at that time would not allow them to indulge in ale or spirits, and wages rising, it may be thought that this practice would cease; but as I do not readily believe that any man having once tasted the divine luxuries of opium will afterwards descend to the gross and mortal enjoyments of alcohol, I take it for granted:
>
> *That those eat now who never ate before;*
> *And those who always ate, now eat the more.*

The number of patent medicines continued to grow, and de Quincey was just one of many Victorians who experimented with and became addicted to opium, often after taking it initially for medicinal purposes. A central character in Wilkie Collins' book *The Moonstone* is a laudanum addict, reflecting the author's own personal experience. The Prime Minister William Gladstone's sister took opium for pain relief and then became hopelessly addicted; he himself took opium before big speeches to settle his nerves. Yet for a long time Victorian society seemed curiously unconcerned that opium-containing medicines were used so indiscriminately. It became rather more pre-occupied with 'opium dens', which were seen as the poisonous influence of foreign cultures. Many famous literary writers of the period described these establishments, including Kipling, Wilde, and Dickens. In the Sherlock Holmes story *The Man with the Twisted Lip* (1892), Arthur Conan Doyle describes an opium den in London's East End. Dr Watson bravely ventures in:

> I found the latch and made my way into a long, low room, thick and heavy with the brown opium smoke, and terraced with wooden berths, like the forecastle of an emigrant ship.
>
> Through the gloom one could dimly catch a glimpse of bodies lying in strange fantastic poses, bowed shoulders, bent knees, heads thrown back, and chins pointing upward, with here and there a dark, lack-lustre eye turned upon the newcomer. Out of the black shadows there glimmered little red circles of light, now bright, now faint, as the burning poison waxed or waned in the bowls of the metal pipes. The most lay silent, but some muttered to themselves, and others talked together in a strange, low, monotonous voice, their conversation coming in gushes, and then suddenly tailing off into silence, each mumbling out

A sketch of a London opium den in 1890. Note that none of the smokers are Europeans.

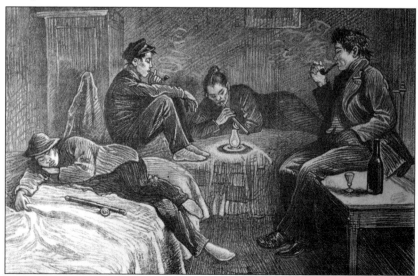

his own thoughts and paying little heed to the words of his neighbour. At the farther end was a small brazier of burning charcoal, beside which on a three-legged wooden stool there sat a tall, thin old man, with his jaw resting upon his two fists, and his elbows upon his knees, staring into the fire.

As I entered, a sallow Malay attendant had hurried up with a pipe for me and a supply of the drug, beckoning me to an empty berth.

In reality, opium dens seem to have been something of a rarity in Britain, and were mainly frequented by those with pre-existing experience of smoking opium – often Asian immigrants or seamen. Nonetheless, inappropriate opium use seems to have been widespread and often indiscriminate.

Overdose and Poisoning

When a very potent drug is widely available and used freely there is always the danger of overdose – either deliberately, with suicidal intent, or accidentally because the patient takes too much by mistake. Children are very sensitive to opium and relatively small amounts can prove fatal, so when curious young fingers found Daddy's opium bottle there were sometimes fatal consequences. Alarmingly, some children's medicines contained opium too and parents might inadvertently give their child an overdose by giving too large a dose or giving it too often. Fatal opium overdose essentially puts the victim to sleep and then stops them breathing, or causes them to vomit and choke on it.

Again, it is surprising perhaps to find an excellent description of opium poisoning in Mrs Beeton's *Book of Household Management*, reflecting that this was a not uncommon domestic problem on account of opium's easy availability. She goes on to recommend how poisoning should be treated:

Give an emetic draught directly, with large quantities of warm mustard-and-water, warm salt-and-water, or simple warm water. Tickle the top of the throat with a feather, or put two fingers down it to bring on vomiting, which rarely takes place by itself. Dash cold water on the head, chest, and spine, and flap these parts well with the ends of wet towels. Give strong coffee or tea. Walk the patient up and down in the open air for two or three hours; the great thing being to keep him from sleeping. Electricity is of much service. When the patient is recovering, mustard poultices should be applied to the soles of the feet and the insides of the thighs and legs. The head should be kept cool and raised.

Wars and Regulation

Opium was so widely used around the world that it became important to British trade. The country even went to war twice over opium. The so-called Opium Wars (1839–42 and 1856–60), arose because Britain wanted to protect its very profitable business in exporting opium from India to China. The problem started when the Chinese government, very reasonably, sought to save its population from an alarming expansion in addiction by banning opium imports. However, Britain saw this as a restriction of trade and declared war, won, then forced China to accept opium imports once more. It was a shameful episode, where a large and powerful country effectively acted like a bullying 'drug lord' to a militarily far weaker nation.

It is a curious irony that shortly after forcing China to sustain its people's addiction, Britain finally passed its first law limiting domestic opium availability because of concerns about over-use in its own citizens. In 1868, the Pharmacy Act confined opium sales to pharmacies – yet this weak law didn't stop abuse and addiction: people merely had fewer outlets from which to obtain opium legally, and the patent medicines were still produced and advertised. It was not until the Dangerous Drugs Act and its regulations in 1920–1 that legislation finally restricted opium to a prescription-only medicine.

Opium cultivation is still the principal source of the morphine used medicinally today, although opium itself is no longer prescribed in Western medicine. Many synthetic morphine-like drugs are now used by doctors instead. It is sobering to appreciate that Heroin was introduced as the brand-name of a morphine derivative which was marketed in 1898 as a *less* addictive form of opium. The rest is, unfortunately, history.

Abuse and Addiction by the Famous

Many eminent eighteenth and nineteenth-century British people are known to have used opium to calm the nerves or to stimulate creativity including Prime Minister William Gladstone, Lord Byron, George IV, Charles Dickens, and Oscar Wilde. Today we would call this drug abuse or recreational drug use, although these terms had no meaning in Victorian times. Several works of fiction are even thought to have been inspired by the effects of opium including *Alice's Adventures in Wonderland* and *The Wizard of Oz*.

Certain leading figures are known to have taken opium short-term for medicinal reasons (e.g. Sir Walter Scott) since it was the only really effective painkiller available. However, other people became long-term users of opium and were in some cases addicted to it. They include Samuel Taylor Coleridge, Wilkie Collins, John Keats, Florence Nightingale, Percy Shelley, and William Wilberforce.

Chapter 17

PLAGUE

The term 'plague' has been used generically in the past to refer to any infectious disease that caused many people to die. Some diseases have even acquired plague-related sobriquets to indicate their virulence – cholera, for example, became known as the 'blue plague' and tuberculosis as the 'white plague'. However, the infection that we today call simply 'plague' was the most potent infectious killer of humans that our species has ever encountered. It has become known by the appropriately sinister name of the Black Death, as well as the bubonic plague.

Plague was caused by bacteria of the species *Yersinia pestis* that infected the fleas living on rats. The fleas hopped off the rats, bit humans to draw blood and in so doing infected them with the bacteria that caused the disease. However, plague can also be transmitted by inhalation of droplets of infected sputum from victims coughing it up into the air.

Symptoms
Certain infectious diseases can be difficult to identify with confidence in historical documents because the symptoms are vague, or might be confused with other illnesses, but this cannot be said of plague because its symptoms are very specific.

The disease started with chills, fever, vomiting, and sometimes sneezing or coughing. Soon afterwards, and usually within three days, the patient developed pain in the groin, armpits, and neck where swellings had developed. These hard, swollen, and painful 'buboes' were characteristic of the disease and could be the size of a large apple. If they burst before the patient died they were found to be filled with pus and left a large ulcer behind. Blisters and carbuncles were additional signs of infection found on the skin, and patients might also bleed from body orifices. The sufferer soon became delirious or confused, lapsed into a comatose state, and then died.

Most people who developed symptoms died – particularly in the early stages of a new epidemic when mortality seems to have been at least 90 per cent. And they died quickly: usually within five or six days of their first symptoms. As an individual epidemic declined, the disease often seemed to become less virulent so that more people began to survive it.

Plague and History

The plague dates back to antiquity, although its earliest documented manifestation is open to doubt. It certainly seems to have existed during the era of classical Greece. The first worldwide outing or pandemic of plague was during the reign of the Roman emperor Justinian, who was one of the fortunate people who apparently contracted the disease but survived. The 'pestilence' began around the year 540 and killed a substantial proportion of the population of the Mediterranean. Plague returned many times during the ensuing years, but seems to have died out in Europe in the eighth century.

After a long lull, the plague returned to Europe. In 1348 it struck the British Isles and this is the principal pandemic now referred to as the Black Death, although the melodramatic name is not a contemporary one – having being invented in the nineteenth century. Plague affected the whole of Europe at this time, where it killed around a third of the entire population, although estimates vary. The effect of so much death on the populace is hard to convey, still harder to relate to in our twenty-first-century world.

The plague traditionally entered fourteenth-century England via the Dorset port of Weymouth, then known as Melcombe. The *Grey Friar's Chronicle* notes:

> In this year 1348 in Melcombe in the county of Dorset, a little before the feast of St John the Baptist, two ships, one of them from Bristol, came alongside. One of the sailors had brought with him from Gascony the seeds of a terrible pestilence and, through him, the men of that town of Melcombe were the first to be infected.

The plague was seen by many as the vengeance of God meted out on his sinful and ungrateful creation. This led people to pray for deliverance from the 'great pestilence', although the more practically minded simply fled. The rapid build-up of corpses meant that it became difficult to deal with them all: individual burial in coffins was in many areas soon abandoned in favour of mass graves. Clergymen who ministered to the dying came into contact with a great many infected persons, and so were particularly badly affected by the disease and they died in disproportionately large numbers.

Many people thought it was the end of the world. There is a very poignant description of the plague in the Kilkenny district of Ireland by a monk, John Clyn, in his *Annals of Ireland*, 1349:

> The pestilence was so contagious that whosoever touched the sick or the dead was immediately infected and died; and the penitent and the confessor were carried together to the grave. Through fear and dread, men scarcely dared to perform the offices of piety and pity in visiting the sick and in burying the dead. Many died of boils and abscesses, and pustules on their shins or under their armpits; others died frantic with the pain in their head, and others spitting blood ...
>
> Scarcely one alone ever died in a house. Commonly husband, wife, children, and servants went the one way – the way of death. And I, Friar John Clyn, of the Order of Friars Minor and of the convent of Kilkenny, wrote in this book these notable things which happened in my time, which I saw with my eyes or which I learned from persons worthy of credit. And lest things worthy of remembrance should perish with time and fall away from the memory of those who are to come after us ... so I have reduced these things to writing, and lest the writing should perish with the writer, and the work fail together with the workman, I leave parchment for continuing the work, if haply any man survive, and any of the race of Adam escape this pestilence and continue the work which I have commenced.

Chillingly, one paragraph later another hand has written: 'Here it seems the author died'.

In Britain, it's tempting to simply focus on this infamous epidemic that began in 1348, and then the well-known Great Plague of London in 1665. However, that would be a mistake. These two outbreaks were effectively historical bookends to the continual presence of plague in this country. It waxed and it waned, killing more people in some years than in others, but it stayed here killing millions of our ancestors for over three centuries.

The plague died down in the early 1350s but saw significant resurgences every few years thereafter until the seventeenth century. These became known as 'plague years'. There were two particularly severe outbreaks in the 1470s, for example; other particularly bad years

– if the death toll in London is anything to go by – included 1592, 1603, 1625, and 1636. After the first outbreak in 1348, the succeeding ones appear to have killed fewer people, presumably because humans were beginning to acquire some resistance to the disease. The disease did not completely go away in the intervening time between plague years; it continued to kill people but simply at a very, very much lower rate. The graph below is based on the reported deaths from plague in London in the seventeenth century, and illustrates the variation in death rate between plague years and non-plague years.

The last major manifestation in Britain was the Great Plague of London which started in 1665 and dissipated in 1666, although this outbreak was not confined to the capital. During the height of the plague, Samuel Pepys, the diarist, wrote to his friend Lady Carteret about his life in London:

> I have stayed in the City till above 7,400 died in one week and of them above 6,000 of the plague, and little noise heard day nor night but the tolling of bells; till I could walk Lombard Street and not meet twenty persons from one end to the other, and not fifty upon the Exchange; till whole families (ten and twelve together) have been swept away; till my very physician, Dr Burnett, who undertook to secure me against infection, died himself of the plague.

Mortality statistics for London 1603–70, showing the percentage attributable to plague each year.

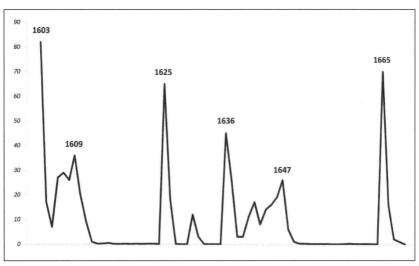

The Bills of Mortality for London in 1665 show that of the 97,306 burials in the city that year, some 68,596 were victims of the plague. These figures represent the officially notified cases and some under-reporting is known to have occurred. In the 1666 Bills of Mortality there were a further 1,998 victims of plague in London, but in subsequent years a few cases only – with the last ever casualties being recorded in 1679.

Once it died out completely, the plague fortunately never returned to these shores in epidemic proportions.

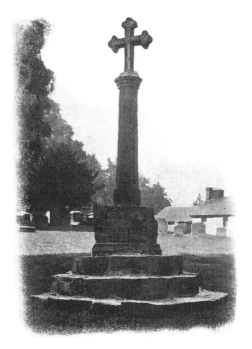

The Plague Cross in Ross-on-Wye, Herefordshire, commemorates a mass grave of 315 plague victims from 1637.

Chapter 18

PREGNANCY AND CHILDBIRTH

Thankfully, most of us can't even begin to imagine how awful it must be when a woman dies after giving birth because these days it is such a rare event. All those months of hope and excitement during pregnancy, the agony of giving birth, and then the horrible realisation that the joy of bringing a baby into the world will be at the expense of its mother's life. Few family events are as tragic as this but sadly most family historians will discover cases of this kind during their research.

The women concerned were usually young, fit, and well before becoming pregnant, and it affected mothers-to-be in all walks of life. Jane Seymour (1508–37), third wife of Henry VIII, died after giving birth to his only legitimate son, the future Edward VI. Henry VIII also lost his mother Elizabeth of York in a similar manner. British statesman Joseph Chamberlain lost both of his wives after childbirth – Harriet in 1863 and Florence, mother of future Prime Minister Neville Chamberlain, in 1875.

In the eighteenth and early nineteenth centuries, death following childbirth was quite common: as many as one or two women dying for every hundred babies born. By the 1850s this had been reduced to

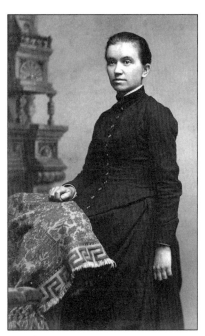

Pregnancy could put a woman's life at risk.

around 1 in 200, and by the 1950s 1 in 1800. Women tend to be more likely to die after giving birth when there is a lack of hygiene, poor nutrition, and inadequate healthcare. These factors also increase infant mortality. Yet if these basic issues are addressed, the number of women dying is dramatically reduced.

Three Main Causes

When researching your ancestry, the only clue to a woman dying as a consequence of giving birth may be the short time interval between the arrival of her baby and the mother's death. This is particularly true before civil registration of deaths began, since parish registers and gravestones are then the most commonly used sources of information about the deceased and they do not generally record causes. Death certificates will usually specify the medical details, but the specialist language used may need some de-coding. There were three principal causes of death: infection, toxaemia, and bleeding.

Infection was the commonest reason for mothers to die after delivery. In particular, puerperal fever was feared because it seemed to occur unpredictably in women who had had a normal, healthy labour. It accounted for as many as half of all maternal deaths before the late Victorian era. We now know that puerperal fever is caused by an infection of the uterus (womb). Doctors, midwives, and their instruments were the unwitting cause of the spread of the disease, and although some early nineteenth-century doctors suggested this, their evidence was ignored. Infection became much less common in the twentieth century when hygiene was understood and antiseptics were widely used.

Puerperal fever began within a few days of giving birth but sometimes might take a week or more to appear. It was not always fatal but most women who died, did so within four weeks of delivery. Some apparently healthy women could die within a week of the onset of symptoms. It started with a fever and as the infection spread it led to septicaemia (blood infection) and/or peritonitis (infection of the abdomen). Women often became delirious before they died: slipping in and out of consciousness, with vivid illusions, and talking incoherently. Those with peritonitis could suffer the most agonising pains – their belly so bloated and sore in some cases that they could not even bear the touch of the bedclothes. Nathaniel Hulme reported this case of puerperal fever and peritonitis in his *A Treatise on the Puerperal Fever*, 1775:

> The patient had an easy labour, and this was her second lying-
> in. The pains were severe all over the lower part of the

abdomen, which was affected by the slightest touch, but particularly in the right iliac region [groin]. A looseness attended from the beginning, and the discharge [diarrhoea] was fetid [it smelt bad]. A vomiting also came on at the same time. Both purging and vomiting continued to the last. The pulse from the first was at one hundred and thirty-six and weak, and before she died, so quick and small as scarcely to be numbered. There was a difficulty in breathing, owing she said, to the acute pain in the abdomen, which was greatly increased every time she drew in her breath. The tongue was white and there was much thirst, and fever. She had a pain in her head and could get no rest. She was strongly prepossessed with a notion, for a long time before her delivery, that she should die in childbed. There was no hiccup, neither was she delirious, but retained her mental faculties perfectly to the time of her death. The disease proved mortal on the seventh day after delivery. [Edited.]

Isabella Beeton is best known for her *Book of Household Management*, but it is less well known that she died of puerperal fever after the birth of her fourth child, aged only 28.

Bleeding was the second well-established killer of women after giving birth, and accounted for around 20 per cent of deaths in the nineteenth century. Although women could survive quite heavy blood loss it could also be a horribly dramatic and rapid way to die, causing great panic amongst all those present when the blood flow could not be stemmed. An important cause was the placenta ('after birth') not being expelled quickly enough when the baby was born. Normally the womb contracts after birth to stop the mother bleeding, but a retained placenta gets in the way. Another cause was tugging on the baby's birth cord too soon after delivery. Bleeding can also happen because of injuries to the womb by it rupturing or being damaged by medical instruments. Whereas most women with an infection took at least a week to die, those dying within 24 hours of delivery usually died due to blood loss.

Mothers could also bleed to death *before* giving birth if the placenta began to come away early (called 'abruption'), or if the placenta blocked the birth canal so that the baby could not be delivered ('placenta praevia').

The third common cause of death was toxaemia, which was responsible for around 10–15 per cent of mothers' deaths. Its precise cause is uncertain but it usually began in the last few weeks of pregnancy and was heralded by a rise in blood pressure, then tiredness, blurred vision, and headache. Following these warning signs, the mother could have fits which proved fatal in around a quarter of those who experienced them. Survivors of fitting might succumb to damage to major organs such as the kidneys, liver, and brain (stroke), which killed some women.

Other Causes

There were a number of other causes of maternal deaths aside from the 'big three' discussed above. Before the twentieth century, lack of vitamin D in the diet caused rickets (see Chapter 9) and this was quite common, especially in Scotland. Rickets caused some women to have distorted bones in the hip area (the pelvis) so that they could not give birth. In these cases women (and their babies) might die in labour.

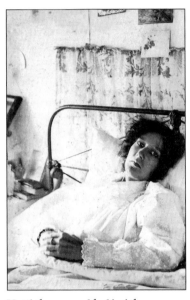

Unfortunately, in former times maternity hospitals and society as a whole encouraged women to rest for weeks after giving birth. This inactivity made blood clots more likely and was responsible for the deaths of some women. Appropriately enough, maternity hospitals were formerly called 'lying-in' hospitals.

Until the second half of the twentieth century, women were expected to rest for many weeks before and after giving birth.

Finally, small numbers of women developed a form of severe mental illness after giving birth. In one form, mothers showed abnormally excitable behaviour, and could turn shockingly violent or abusive. In another form, women became very depressed. Some of these women recovered, but others died – sometimes through suicide – or were put into lunatic asylums.

The Aftermath

The most immediate concern of the husband, beyond attending to his own grief, was the care of his newborn baby if it survived and any other children he had. In the short term, female relatives were often willing to assist him with day-to-day care, and you will often find that the man's sister or mother temporarily moves into the family home for this purpose. Sometimes this is picked up via the census. Wet nurses were also an option for newborn babies: these women were paid to breastfeed other people's infants.

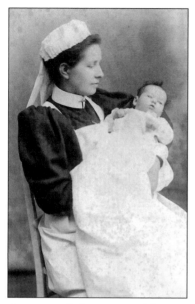

A nanny or infant nurse might care for a baby in richer families.

Often the widower and his family would soon set about looking for a potential new wife to take on the maternal responsibilities of the household. This haste to re-marry may look unseemly to us, since men in this situation often did re-marry quickly, yet in practical terms the husband's re-marriage was usually an economic and familial necessity. In former times, men were the breadwinners and they could not earn an income if they were at home caring for children. Nannies, an infant nurse, or servants were an option for the better off, but most families could not afford them. Considerate employers might permit a husband a brief period of absence from work, but self-employed men and those on low incomes could allow themselves only a brief respite because not working meant no income.

It was often the case that a man would re-marry someone already known to the family – ideally a spinster or a woman who had herself been widowed. Women who already had several children by a former marriage were not an attractive economic prospect for men who already had to provide for children of their own.

Abortion

In a discussion of deaths after childbirth, it is important not to overlook the many women who died by choosing to end their pregnancy early because their baby was not wanted. Before abortion was legalised in England, Wales, and Scotland, illegal abortions could be procured to terminate a pregnancy. Some were performed by pregnant women themselves, some by midwives and doctors, and others by non-medically qualified 'backstreet' abortionists. Practices were often crude and dangerous. Popular methods included taking very hot baths, inducing accidents (e.g. throwing oneself downstairs), various forms of physical invasion of the womb, and the taking of a variety of drugs, plants, and poisons.

In the 1930s, there were around 44,000 illegal abortions in England and Wales, and maybe as many as 3–5 per cent of these caused the mother to die, usually because of infection. On a death certificate it may be disguised with a different diagnosis to protect the reputation of the family. The women who sought abortions were not necessarily unmarried young women who were unaware of the 'facts of life' or those with many male partners; there was a high proportion of older women for whom the primitive methods of contraception then available had failed.

After 1938, a legal ruling permitted a medical abortion in restricted circumstances: when two doctors agreed that a woman's physical or mental health would be impaired by pregnancy. As of 2012, this is still substantially the legal position in Northern Ireland, but for England, Wales, and Scotland the Abortion Act of 1967 rendered abortion legal during the first twenty-eight weeks of pregnancy, although this was reduced to twenty-four weeks in 1990.

Twenty-first Century

Mercifully, a mother dying as a result of giving birth is now very rare in Britain thanks to better knowledge of hygiene, improved obstetric and midwifery techniques, antenatal care and monitoring during pregnancy, and our ability to prevent and treat maternal illness. In 2008 the number of mothers dying as a result of childbirth stood at only 1 case in every 12,200 births in Britain. Sadly, however, in parts of the Third World such as central Africa and Afghanistan, the incidence is similar to Britain 150 years ago: a shocking 1 in 63.

Your Ancestors and Death in Childbirth

As already mentioned, a short interval between the child's birth and the mother dying is highly suggestive of birth-related death. This is important because sometimes the causes cited on Victorian death certificates can be rather vague (e.g. 'fever'). Confusingly, the medical profession has often failed to agree on precise names for maternal illnesses so there are many variants, with some terms changing their meaning over the years. Some examples are given below:

- Puerperal fever – recorded as childbed or womb fever, metria, puerperal sepsis, puerperal infection, puerperal peritonitis, puerperal metritis, postpartum sepsis, postpartum pyaemia, endometritis, and pelvic abscess.
- Toxaemia – has been known as eclampsia, pre-eclampsia, eclamptic fits, puerperal convulsions, puerperal nephritis with albuminuria, and hypertensive disease of pregnancy.

- Bleeding after delivery – postpartum haemorrhage, retained placenta, and flooding. Bleeding before delivery was called accidental haemorrhage, placental abruption, or placenta praevia.
- Blood clots – might be referred to as deep-vein thrombosis, phlegmasia dolens, puerperal arteritis, milk leg, pulmonary embolus, or sudden death.
- Severe mental illness after birth – has been called puerperal insanity, puerperal mania, and puerperal psychosis. Where depression happens this is called postpartum (or postnatal) depression or melancholia.

Chapter 19

SCURVY

Anyone who went to sea for prolonged periods before 1900 would have been all too familiar with scurvy. It was a much-feared illness, particularly in the eighteenth century, and was caused by inadequate vitamin C in the diet. Even today, the chemical name for vitamin C is ascorbic acid, with 'ascorbic' meaning 'without scurvy'. In the era before its cause was known, scurvy was fatal unless the sufferer happened to eat some food containing the vitamin. During his 1741 circumnavigation of the globe, Commodore Anson lost a staggering two-thirds of his 2,000 crew – mostly due to scurvy.

A Sea Disease?

Although usually thought of as a 'sea disease', scurvy did affect land dwellers. It was seen in situations where people were denied a balanced diet for a long time such as in besieged towns, prison populations, and in communities or individuals surviving at subsistence level. It also came about when armies on prolonged campaign abroad were supplied with inadequate rations (e.g. in the Crimea).

Scurvy's association with the sea arose because during the eighteenth century a large naval fleet was needed to patrol the extensive British possessions overseas. This required long voyages, protracted campaigns, and a continuous naval presence often over periods of years. Accordingly, the number of ships and seamen grew enormously and men spent very long periods at sea – sometimes years. By 1799, the navy operated more than 800 ships and employed over 125,000 fighting men. Despite almost continuous warfare in the eighteenth century, in which the Royal Navy was heavily involved, scurvy is believed to have killed many more sailors than Britain's wartime enemies.

The standard Royal Navy ship's fare in the eighteenth century consisted of food that would withstand prolonged storage. The diet was principally salted meat (usually pork or beef), dried peas, cereals such as

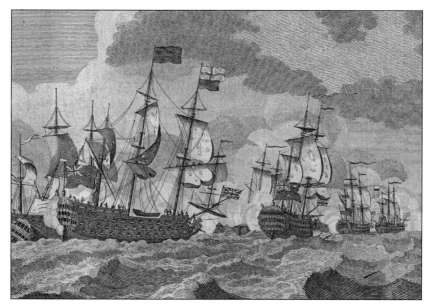

Royal Navy ships in 1760. Scurvy killed thousands of their crews every year.

oatmeal, ship's biscuits, butter, and cheese. This was all washed down with beer and rum, or water if alcoholic drinks were not available. None of these foods or beverages contain a significant amount of vitamin C. A ship might occasionally take on a supply of root vegetables or fruit such as apples which do contain small amounts of the vitamin, but these were soon eaten. Officers fared better than seamen because they could afford to supplement their navy rations with food of good quality which they brought with them or purchased when the ship entered a port. They were also able to obtain regular shore leave and so eat a more balanced diet intermittently.

Symptoms

The symptoms of scurvy were well known to every seaman. The most obvious initial sign was swelling and bleeding of the gums, bad breath, and a spotty complexion. Sufferers then began to become lethargic, and wounds refused to heal – indeed wounds that had healed many years previously could suddenly burst open again. Scurvy affected the immune system as well, which rendered victims prone to infections. Consequently, men who ostensibly died from wound infections or 'fever' had, in many cases, often succumbed because deprivation of vitamin C had weakened their ability to fend off infection. Ultimately, scurvy made those affected feel so mentally drained and physically weak that they were unable even to stand up on board ship, let alone carry out their duties or respond to orders. Some people became delirious or suffered hallucinations before they died.

Using the prevailing eighteenth-century approach to investigating disease, doctors sought the cause of scurvy by examining the *environment* in which it was contracted and the *behaviour* of those who suffered from it. A popular theory was that scurvy was caused by over-exposure to cold, damp sea air. Others blamed the notorious sexual promiscuity of sailors. Yet recognising that lethargy was a significant symptom, another curiously persistent proposal was that scurvy was caused by sailors being lazy or having an inappropriate mental attitude: after all, seamen frequently had to be encouraged to obey orders – and sometimes punished – yet officers, who were more motivated and diligent, didn't tend to contract scurvy.

By the 1740s there were a variety of popular treatments for scurvy. Preparations containing a waterside plant called 'scurvy grass' were popular, as were those containing orange juice – both of which contain vitamin C – but there were many ineffective treatments peddled for profit at sufferers' expense. Oranges, lemon juice, and fruit generally, had been advocated by various people for a couple of centuries or more, yet with so many other useless treatments around, no one knew which were truly effective. The navy had favoured a variety of curious treatments including the drinking of sulphuric acid, cider, seawater, malt drinks, or vinegar; fumigation with burning sulphur or washing the ship with vinegar; and the taking of various patent medicines. Ventilating the ship to relieve its stale atmosphere below decks was also advocated. A bizarre treatment favoured by some was to bury affected seamen up to their necks in sand.

James Lind

In 1747, James Lind, ship's surgeon on HMS *Salisbury*, selected twelve men with similar scurvy symptoms for what has been described as the world's first clinical trial. He tried six different treatments one of which was 'two oranges and one lemon given them every day', and compared all six treatments with each other, as well as with a group of men ('controls') given no treatments. The effects were remarkable – the two men given citrus fruits improved dramatically within six days: one returned to duty, the other stayed to nurse the remaining ten who showed no significant improvements, even after fourteen days' treatment. Here was proof at last that citrus fruit – and the vitamin C they contained – cured scurvy. Lind published a treatise explaining his findings and sent it to the Admiralty.

He expanded his treatise when he became surgeon in charge of the Royal Navy Hospital at Haslar, where he administered the remedy to all scurvy sufferers. Lind soon realised that taking large quantities of lemon juice could cause stomach pain. He thus advised starting with small doses and mixing the juice with other substances such as sugar and wine to dilute it.

In a later edition of his *Treatise on the Scurvy*, originally published in 1753, Lind summarised his extensive clinical experience of treating scurvy victims:

> To what has already been said of the virtues of oranges and lemons in this disease, I have now to add that in seemingly the most desperate cases, the most quick and sensible relief was obtained from lemon juice; by which I have relieved many hundred patients, labouring under almost intolerable pain and affliction from this disease, when no other remedy seemed to avail. And particularly at Haslar Hospital, where the scurvy raged in the year 1759, many, with whom the distemper increased during a course of other medicines, and a plentiful diet of green vegetables, owed their recovery entirely to the lemon juice.

Unhappily, the Admiralty did not act on Lind's findings largely because this was an era when society was unused to making important decisions based on scientific evidence. There were too many competing 'cures' for scurvy – many with their own powerful advocates within the navy – and the Admiralty lacked the ability to discriminate between them logically. Lind also lacked the ability to push his findings more forcefully. Captains who cured their men's scurvy by buying citrus fruits whilst in foreign ports were made to pay for them themselves.

The Cure Available

It was not until 1799 that citrus juice was made generally available to all navy ships, and that was thanks largely to the persistence of another surgeon, Gilbert Blane. Regrettably, James Lind did not live to see his research put into practice. Lemon juice was a simple remedy, but it made all the difference.

However, despite Admiralty instructions it took some time for them to come fully into effect – surgeons sometimes reserving citrus juices to treat cases of scurvy rather than administering it regularly to the whole crew to prevent the disease. In 1802, William Cather, surgeon on HMS *Vanguard*, wrote in his Surgeon's Journal:

Remarks about scurvy cases

from the 12th or 14th day from the first attack, most of them complained of giddiness and sickness at stomach, and from the slightest exertion they frequently have fainted about this time also, the face became cadaverous, with great debility, loss of appetite. As the lividness in the lower extremities increased, those parts became as tense – as hard almost as a board. In two cases the back of the hand only was affected.

Treatment

About this time we were lucky in procuring from an American ship, a few bags of onions, which were given me for the use of the scorbuticks [scurvy sufferers], and they were ordered to eat them raw with vinegar, the bowels in all being previously gently opened. They also took the bark and lime juice four times a day, of which I had plenty and I gave them lemonade *ad libitum* besides, they had a mess of portable soup with barley, with the other comforts which the necessaries afford; by these means we kept the disease from gaining much upon us, nor did we lose a man, although when we arrived at Halifax I had ill of scurvy 113.

[ADM 101/124/2 at TNA]

Nonetheless, the administration of citrus juices on board navy ships gradually made an impact: there were nearly 1,500 cases of scurvy admitted to the Royal Navy hospital at Haslar in 1780; in 1809 there were none.

Men serving in the merchant navy were at reduced risk of scurvy because their time at sea was much less than for navy men, and their diet was probably better. Nonetheless, men on long foreign voyages could still be badly affected. Unlike the navy, however, there was no single employer who could act, so legislation was required. Yet this didn't happen until 1851 and because so many vessels didn't comply, it had to be strengthened by additional legislation, the Merchant Shipping Act of 1867:

The master of every [foreign-going] ship as last aforesaid shall serve or cause to be served out the lime or lemon juice with sugar or other such anti-scorbutics as aforesaid to the crew so soon as they have been at sea for ten days, and during the

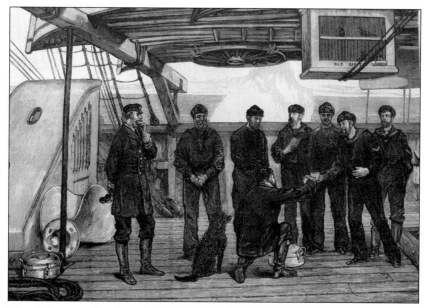

Lime juice served on board a Royal Navy ship in 1875.

remainder of the voyage, except during such time as they are in harbour and are there supplied with fresh provisions; the lime or lemon juice and sugar to be served out daily at the rate of an ounce each per day to each member of the crew, and to be mixed with a due proportion of water before being served out, or the other anti-scorbutics, if any, at such times and in such quantities as Her Majesty by order in council may from time to time direct.

This Act protecting the health of merchant seamen was passed some 120 years after Lind's clinical trial.

At some point following the recommendation to use lemon juice, it became acceptable to use lime juice instead and some companies produced this in a preserved form – including the famous Rose's Lime Cordial. This later led to British seamen being referred to as 'limeys' by their American counterparts. Unfortunately, lime juice contains less vitamin C than lemon juice and, besides, some juices were of poor quality and contained insufficient vitamin. In other situations citrus juices were available on board but not given. In one infamous case in 1875, a British expedition to the Arctic resulted in men not receiving lime juice after they had left their ship. Two-thirds of the crew on board HMS *Alert* suffered severe scurvy and many were incapacitated in the snowy wastes; two men died.

A parliamentary report highlighted the resurgence of scurvy: there had been only twenty-two outbreaks of scurvy in British ships in 1869, but in 1881 there were ninety-nine. It recommended that a more effective preventive was the adoption of a better diet. This gradually led to seamen receiving a more balanced diet at sea and the scurvy problem eventually abated.

Your Ancestors and Scurvy

Cause of death in the eighteenth-century navy was typically only recorded in the ship's log if it occurred as a result of an accident (e.g. 'fell overboard'), or a naval engagement ('killed in action'). In other situations the cause of death is often not given or is vague (e.g. 'fever'). However, senior officers' correspondence may provide a clue that an ancestor died of scurvy since they often wrote about the general state of their crews in terms of preparedness for battle. For example, Vice Admiral Hughes wrote to the Admiralty concerning his squadron in 1783:

> So early as the 8th of June, the scurvy began to make a rapid progress among the crews of all the ships of the squadron, but particularly on board the ships last arrived from England. The number of sick on board the line of battle ships amounted on that day to 1,121 men, 605 of whom being in the last stage of the scurvy. From the 22nd, the disease increased the numbers of the sick daily, so as most of the ships of the line had from 70 to 90 men, and the ships last from England double that number, very many in the last stage of the disease, and unable to come to quarters, dying daily. [Edited; reproduced in Charles Ekins' *Naval Battles of Great Britain*, 1829.]

Sadly these men and many others died quite unnecessarily, over thirty-five years after Lind had proved that lemon juice could have saved them.

The records associated with naval hospitals such as Haslar may also contain evidence of scurvy amongst patients. From the late 1790s onwards the logs of ships' surgeons usually record illness fairly precisely, and many of these cases are indexed by seaman's name in TNA's online Discovery service.

In contemporary records, scurvy was sometimes known as scorbie, *purpura nautica*, blacklegs, the Dutch distemper, or *scorbutus*. Medications used to treat scurvy were referred to as anti-scorbutics.

Chapter 20

SMALLPOX

The smallpox was always present, filling the churchyards with corpses, tormenting with constant fears all whom it had not yet stricken, leaving on those whose lives it spared the hideous traces of its power, turning the babe into a changeling at which the mother shuddered, and making the eyes and cheeks of the betrothed maiden objects of horror to the lover.

Thomas Macaulay, *The History of England*, 1848

Smallpox is a disease unique to humans and may have originated in Africa since the oldest known case is an Egyptian pharaoh's mummy from 1500 BCE. In Europe, this infection began to become much more common during the seventeenth century, probably because urbanisation provided greater concentrations of people to act upon. By the end of the eighteenth century, it has been estimated that smallpox was killing as many as 400,000 Europeans every year, and children were the main victims.

Heavily populated areas were particularly badly affected since smallpox was highly contagious, and the cramped conditions of inner cities enabled it to spread quickly. Although the disease was ever-present, there were regular intense outbreaks where many more people than usual were affected. This happened because smallpox could only be spread from one person to the next by people who had never had it before: when they became infected they were also contagious. Survivors were immune to a second attack. People who had never suffered smallpox were generally children, or travellers from areas where smallpox was less common such as the countryside. Once enough of these susceptible people had built up in a population, an outbreak would occur and run rampant through them. These epidemics developed suddenly, spread very rapidly, and then disappeared quickly after just a few weeks. Understandably, smallpox was highly feared.

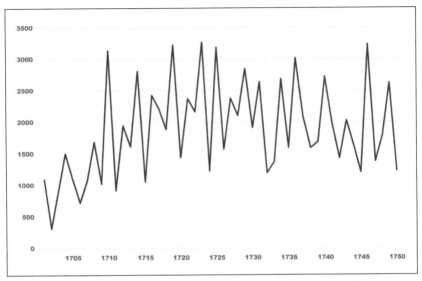

Annual numbers of smallpox fatalities in London 1700–50. Outbreaks every two or three years caused deaths to peak.

The fluctuating death rate from the disease was most striking in cities such as London where there were regular epidemics every two to three years. In rural areas it took much longer for a nucleus of susceptible people to build up – mainly because there were fewer children than in large towns – so the epidemics tended to strike less frequently (e.g. every five to seven years).

Not everyone infected with smallpox died, but as many as one in every five deaths in the eighteenth century was due directly or indirectly to the illness. The majority of these were children. Sadly, many family historians will be familiar with parish registers during this period recording large numbers of infant and childhood deaths, and smallpox was the principal cause.

Scottish doctor William Cullen reported a poignant case that he attended which highlights the suddenness with which victims could surrender to the illness:

> Mrs Squires of Northfleet, in the last month of her pregnancy, in the year 1780, was on the Thursday or Friday taken with fever and its usual attendants; on the Saturday she was delivered. About two hours after delivery the small-pox appeared, was very full and of the coherent kind. She died on the Friday. The child died the Tuesday week following, having lived nine days;

it might have died in one of those fits which frequently precede the eruption of the small-pox.

Symptoms

Smallpox was caused by a virus, and was also known as variola – not to be confused with 'varicella', which is another name for chickenpox. It was exhaled in the breath of infected people and in this form it was highly contagious, so close contact with sufferers allowed the virus to spread rapidly. The first symptoms were fever, headache, chills, and vomiting which intensified over the course of a few days, sometimes causing children to fit.

After about three days a distinctive rash appeared and covered the whole body, but was more concentrated on the face, and the lower ends of the limbs. It started as tiny red spots but quickly developed into large, hard, painful pimples called 'pocks' with a small hollow pit at the top of each one, surrounded by red inflammation. The face often swelled dramatically as these pocks grew and many sufferers could not even open their eyes. Often there were so many pocks that they all ran together covering large areas of the skin and this 'confluent' form was much more likely to be fatal. After about a week the pocks burst.

About one in three people died from smallpox – usually during the first two weeks. Almost all survivors experienced facial scarring after the pocks scabbed and fell off. The pitted scars were permanent and in many cases, disfiguring. Smallpox was also the leading cause of blindness in eighteenth-century Europe.

The disease spread so rapaciously that by the end of the eighteenth century it would probably be true to say that all our adult ancestors then living were smallpox survivors. Many other contagious infections such as plague, TB and cholera affected poor people disproportionately because they lived in crowded unsanitary conditions. However, smallpox spread so easily that it affected all sections of society equally. It has often been noted, for example, that several significant European monarchs were killed by the disease including Louis XV of France (1774), Queen Ulrika of Sweden (1741), Tsar Peter II of Russia (1730), and Mary II of England (1694).

Edward Jenner

Since the early eighteenth century there had been a means to prevent the worst effects of smallpox. A technique called variolation or inoculation involved scratching the skin and deliberately infecting it with pus from the pocks of someone with a less severe form of smallpox. The aim was to induce a mild case of smallpox which would make the affected person immune to it. However, variolation carried risks since some people developed full-blown smallpox, and up to 2 per cent of them died as a result. This technique had been known about for many years outside Europe, but probably began in England and Wales in the early eighteenth century where it was taken up by many, but not universally.

The *Memoirs of the Royal Society* from 1740 recorded what already seemed common practice:

> In Wales, the custom of 'buying the smallpox', as it is called, is a common practice and of long standing. The manner of communicating the infectious matter to the blood is by scraping the skin with a penknife, and so rubbing in the matter. Mr Owen bought the smallpox when at school and gave threepence for the matter contained in 12 pustules. It is certain that hundreds in this country have had the small-pox this way, and not one single instance can be produced of their ever having them a second time. [Edited.]

Later it was recognised that farmworkers who contracted a disease of cattle called 'cowpox' also became resistant to smallpox. Indeed, in 1774, a Dorset farmer, Benjamin Jesty, claimed that his wife and two sons never contracted smallpox after he performed a variolation-type technique on them with cowpox instead of smallpox.

A country doctor, Edward Jenner, took all this work a stage further by providing scientific proof that exposing people to cowpox prevented smallpox. In May 1796 he took matter from a cowpox pustule on the finger of a dairymaid called Sarah Nelmes and inoculated it into the arm of a young boy, James Phipps. Then around seven weeks later he injected him with smallpox. James failed to react to smallpox at all, demonstrating that he was now immune.

Jenner wrote up his experiment and presented it to the Royal Society which refused to publish it, so he published it privately in 1798. He called the cowpox technique 'vaccination', from the Latin word for cow, *vacca*. Jenner managed to convince a sceptical medical profession, initially in London, that vaccination worked and the good news spread rapidly. In 1800 he personally vaccinated the entire 85th Regiment. He helped vaccination to be accepted by governments and peoples all around the world, by supplying samples of cowpox material to doctors from many countries. He received many honours in his lifetime, including payment of £30,000 from a grateful British government. His fame was such that when he petitioned Napoleon to release some British prisoners of war, the Emperor acquiesced to the doctor's request and said: 'Jenner – I can refuse him nothing'.

Jenner wrote to a friend in 1809: 'It will be no news to you that vaccination goes on most charmingly all the world over. The information I derive from all quarters allows me to say that wherever it is universally adopted, the smallpox ceases to exist.'

Campaigners Against Vaccination

Opposition to vaccination is almost as old as vaccination itself, and has found ready media coverage from the nineteenth to the twenty-first centuries. Safety issues have often featured prominently and it is no surprise to learn that even 200 years ago concerns were raised that Jenner's vaccination would turn people into cows. Then, as now, there were religious objections as well – some people believed it was somehow immoral to take organic matter from lowly cows and inject it into people.

Many European countries introduced nationwide vaccination within a few years of Jenner publishing his work. Britain was relatively slow to do this, but the Vaccination Act of 1853 rendered vaccination compulsory.

A ward at Hampstead Smallpox Hospital during the epidemic of the 1870s.

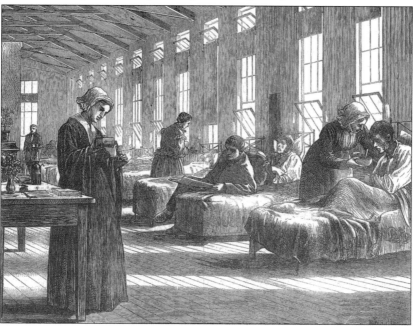

This provoked riots in some English towns, including Ipswich. In London, anti-vaccination organisations arose and acted as a focus for opposition. They argued with alarm that compulsory vaccination was a violation of personal freedom and the right to choose.

The last large-scale smallpox epidemic in Britain was in 1870–3 and killed 44,000 people in England and Wales. This was a better incentive to vaccination than the law, and overrode any qualms that most people might have had: it helped to sustain high vaccination rates during the Victorian era. At the beginning of the outbreak in 1870, the *Illustrated London News* reported from the Hampstead Smallpox Hospital:

[The hospital] is one of four fever and smallpox hospitals in the metropolis under the general management of the Metropolitan Asylums Board. In these four institutions about 24,000 patients in round numbers have been treated during the smallpox epidemic. The patients are admitted to the hospitals on the relieving officer's orders; and though the patients are thus paupers, the parishes are entitled by law, if the persons are able to pay, to recover the cost of their keep in these asylums.

Despite the hard lessons of the 1870s, in 1898 British law was changed so that parents opposed to vaccination could receive exemption certificates for their children.

The Killer Dies

In the twentieth century widescale smallpox vaccination, and rapid quarantine responses to outbreaks as they occurred, began severely to restrict the impact of smallpox. In 1980, the WHO announced that a prediction made by Jenner himself had come true: smallpox was dead. The last naturally occurring human case occurred in Somalia in 1977.

Although two small samples of smallpox virus have been kept alive in research laboratories, smallpox virus no longer exists in nature. This is one of the biggest reasons for the much greater British life expectancy in the twenty-first century compared to two or three centuries ago.

Your Ancestors and Smallpox

As already noted, when parish records list the ages of the deceased they can show large numbers of children dying in a community at the same time and this may be evidence of smallpox. However, since there are many other potential causes (see Chapter 7) sometimes you can get circumstantial evidence for smallpox by scrutinising local newspapers or

The smallpox vaccination certificate for Alice Waller of Hartlepool in 1858.

historical records to see if there was a notable outbreak at the time. For those who died in London in the seventeenth and eighteenth centuries, the annual Bills of Mortality will reveal whether this happened in a year when smallpox was rife. Many of these reports are available on Google Books at http://books.google.com.

If you have pictures of ancestors from Victorian times, then a pitted complexion could be evidence of the scars of a smallpox survivor. Female victims might adopt heavy make-up, beauty spots, and even veils to hide their scars; some men resorted to growing facial hair.

Although not evidence of the disease, you may find that a smallpox vaccination certificate has survived amongst family papers for one of your ancestors. They have quite often been preserved because of the legal penalties for not vaccinating children at the time.

Chapter 21

TROPICAL INFECTIONS

From the sixteenth century onwards, the British started to operate on a world stage. Our ancestors began to find their way to the far reaches of the globe because of voyages of exploration, the growing importance of the sea for trade, colonialism, foreign wars, and emigration. Trans-oceanic travel meant that people would encounter new diseases. West Africa soon acquired notoriety as the 'white man's grave' because so many Europeans died there from mysterious tropical fevers, and the Caribbean was known as the 'fever islands'.

A whole host of tropical diseases might confront the newcomer to the Americas, Africa, and Asia, and one problem for family historians is that illnesses contracted abroad can be described quite loosely by terms such as 'fever'. Eighteenth and nineteenth-century doctors considered that the high temperatures in the tropics, the humidity, and the very bright sun weakened the European constitution. Indeed, some even believed that the tropics were unnatural places for white people to live and that they would never survive there long-term.

Two diseases in particular were to prove widely fatal – yellow fever and malaria. Both were transmitted by mosquitoes. A mosquito looks so insignificant when you brush one away that it is hard to imagine it could be anything more than a nuisance. Yet many of our ancestors died because they were bitten by one.

Yellow Fever
Yellow fever is caused by a virus that probably emerged in Africa about 3,000 years ago. It is injected into humans by the *Aëdes* mosquito when it feeds on people's blood. Most of those who become infected suffer from an influenza-like illness and then recover. Yet one in seven develops much more severe symptoms such as jaundice, pain, and bleeding, and about 20 per cent of these die. The jaundice turns the victim's skin bright yellow, and this led to the disease's name.

In the 1600s yellow fever was carried from Africa to the Americas, probably via slave ships, and caused outbreaks of disease initially amongst the indigenous people. However, in 1668 there was an epidemic in New York, and other eastern American cities followed. It also quickly spread to the Caribbean islands. These are all areas where British people lived and worked.

The almost unending warfare in the eighteenth century meant that European navies repeatedly transported mosquitoes and infected persons from place to place. Although it was soon noticed that outbreaks usually began at seaports, contemporary doctors thought that the

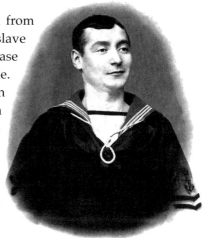

Eighteenth and nineteenth-century sailors often fell victim to yellow fever.

disease was either spread from person to person by contact, or arose spontaneously from the filth and sewage found in docks and harbours.

This constant spreading of disease by ships meant that the Americas and the Caribbean experienced repeated outbreaks of yellow fever throughout the eighteenth century. A particularly notorious one in Philadelphia in 1793 killed an estimated 10 per cent of the population.

British sailors visiting Africa and the Americas became afraid of yellow fever. In Panama, for example, 4,000 Royal Navy seamen succumbed to the disease in 1727 whilst laying siege to the Spanish port of Port Bello. Even in the nineteenth century navy ships continued to lose men to this dread disease on a regular basis. In the early twentieth century, yellow fever killed so many workers that it threatened to prevent completion of the Panama Canal. European colonists and seamen in Africa were particularly liable to this disease and it was noted that whilst native Africans suffered from it, Europeans were much more likely to die.

Fevers were generally treated in the same way in the seventeenth to mid-nineteenth centuries. The unfortunate patients were bled, bathed with cold water, and given medicines to make them vomit or produce diarrhoea. Doctors felt that taking blood, and emptying the bowel, would help remove whatever was causing the fever and restore the body's natural balance. By the same logic, some doctors also gave medicines to promote salivation and sweating. In the nineteenth century, various formulations of 'fever powders' were popular remedies to take by mouth but they were of doubtful efficacy.

It was not until 1881, that Carlos Finlay proposed that yellow fever might be transmitted by mosquitoes and this was soon proved. A mosquito eradication programme in some countries managed completely to eliminate the disease, and the last outbreak in the USA was in 1905. A yellow fever vaccine was developed in the 1930s and this has successfully protected many future generations.

Malaria

Although malaria is now a tropical disease, it used to occur widely in Europe. In Britain it was found mainly in the estuaries and marshes of East Anglia, and south-east and northern England. However, the draining of marshland, climate change, and urbanisation helped to eradicate malaria as a native disease. The last large local outbreak of malaria in Britain was just after the First World War, when returning troops brought infected mosquitoes back with them, and this is believed to have killed up to 500 civilians in Kent. Yet malaria proved more common and more severe when encountered abroad in India, south-east Asia, western Africa, and South America.

Malaria is an ancient disease that pre-dates modern humans. Its association with stagnant, smelly water has been known for over 2,000 years. This is the environment in which the malaria mosquito breeds and lives, but doctors came to believe that malaria was caused by bad air itself: the odour from marshes acting as some kind of poisonous gas or 'miasma'. This idea persisted until the nineteenth century – indeed the word 'malaria' means 'bad air' in Italian.

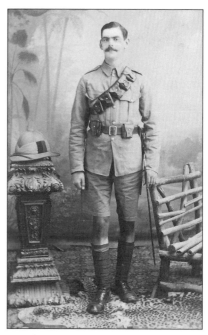

British soldiers serving in India were prone to malaria.

Like yellow fever, malaria also starts with flu-like symptoms but the onset can be delayed for months after the original mosquito bite. The fever may also alternate with periods of chills. Malaria can cause fits, anaemia, breathing problems, blood clots, coma, and death.

In the seventeenth century, Jesuit missionaries in Peru became aware that natives used the bark of the cinchona tree to treat malaria. The bark became known in Europe as 'Peruvian Bark' or 'Jesuit's Bark' and because of its expense it was initially available only to the wealthy. In 1820, the active ingredient of the bark was identified as quinine, which we now know kills the malaria parasite.

By the end of the nineteenth century, quinine was widely used to treat and prevent malaria. Soldiers deployed abroad were commonly dosed with it on a daily basis, but quinine is very bitter so some of them began mixing it with a little sugar and a dash of gin. This is the origin of our modern 'gin and tonic'. Schweppes developed its Indian Tonic Water in the 1870s, and it still contains quinine.

Once the concept of germs causing disease was accepted by the medical profession in the late nineteenth century, then the search began for an organism that caused malaria. Charles Laveran was the first to show that malaria was caused by a parasite called *Plasmodium* in 1880, and this was soon followed by Ronald Ross's discovery that the *Anopheles* mosquito carried the parasite and transmitted the disease.

By the 1930s, malaria was becoming resistant to quinine. As a result new drugs were developed over the course of the twentieth century, including mepacrine, chloroquine, proguanil and mefloquine. These last three are still used.

Twenty-first Century

These days we have tablets to reduce the risk of malaria, mosquito nets, insect repellent sprays, and a vaccine against yellow fever. Despite the fact that both malaria and yellow fever can be prevented, in 2010 there were an estimated 216 million cases of malaria worldwide and 200,000 victims of yellow fever. In Britain we are fortunate that we can call on medical protection when we travel, unlike our ancestors, and unlike many Third World people living today.

Other Tropical Diseases

Leprosy is a very disfiguring bacterial infection that also causes considerable long-term nerve and muscle damage. It was an important disease of medieval Europe where lepers were forced to live apart from unaffected individuals, sometimes in leper colonies. It has become progressively rarer in Europe over the past 200 years, but in the nineteenth century was still a well-known disease amongst those who travelled to tropical areas such as central Africa, India and South America.

There are many other diseases that our ancestors may have encountered when venturing abroad. Some examples include:

- African sleeping sickness (trypanosomiasis) is transmitted by the tsetse fly.
- Amoebic dysentery is spread by poor sanitation.
- Bilharzia (schistosomiasis) and filariasis are caused by small worms invading the body.
- Cholera is caused by poor sanitation, and it spread globally on several occasions in the nineteenth century (see Chapter 8).
- Dengue fever is a viral disease spread by mosquitoes.
- Relapsing fever infects people via ticks or lice.
- Leishmaniasis is spread by sand flies and causes sores on the body.
- River blindness (onchocerciasis) is transmitted by a species of black fly.
- Yaws is an ulcerating infection passed from person to person by contact.

Your Ancestors and Tropical Illness

The alternating fever and chills typical of malaria were often referred to as the 'ague' in contemporary records such as death certificates. Malaria was the disease described by phrases such as blackwater fever, congestive fever, marsh miasm, paludal poison, remitting fever, swamp sickness, or marsh fever. Quartan fever is a less serious form of malaria.

Yellow fever was known as the American plague, black vomit, haemorrhagic fever, bronze John, dock fever, stranger's fever, and yellow jack.

It is not uncommon to find malaria or yellow fever cited as a cause of death on British memorials commemorating the lives of people who died abroad – especially in the services. For example, one at All Saints Church, Great Braxted, records the death of Reginald Evans Grant in 1918 'who contracted malaria at the Battle of Damascus and died at Alexandria'. Similarly, a monument at Southsea commemorates 'Forty-eight officers and men who died during the epidemic of yellow fever on board HMS *Aboukir* at Jamaica in 1873–4'.

Records of the Royal Navy's surgeons 1793–1880, in series ADM 101 at TNA, can be searched by patient's name using http://discovery. nationalarchives.gov.uk. Using advanced search, type in a surname and restrict the 'search within' to series ADM 101. Here you will find all manner of tropical complaints recorded amongst seamen on their travels, including some unusual ones such as being bitten by a shark or stung by a scorpion.

Chapter 22

TUBERCULOSIS

There is a dread disease which so prepares its victim, as it were, for death; which so refines it of its grosser aspect, and throws around familiar looks unearthly indications of the coming change; a dread disease, in which the struggle between soul and body is so gradual, quiet, and solemn, and the result so sure, that day by day, and grain by grain, the mortal part wastes and withers away, so that the spirit grows light and sanguine with its lightening load, and, feeling immortality at hand, deems it but a new term of mortal life; a disease in which death and life are so strangely blended, that death takes the glow and hue of life, and life the gaunt and grisly form of death; a disease which medicine never cured, wealth never warded off, or poverty could boast exemption from; which sometimes moves in giant strides, and sometimes at a tardy sluggish pace, but, slow or quick, is ever sure and certain.

Charles Dickens, *The Life and Adventures
of Nicholas Nickleby*, 1838–9

In Victorian society, as many as one in six people died of tuberculosis – a slowly lethal infection – so it is no coincidence that Dickens brings it to the fore in one of his greatest novels. Between 1700 and 1900, tuberculosis, TB, or the 'white plague' killed an estimated 1 billion people worldwide.

Yet despite its frequency as a cause of death on Victorian death certificates, TB is an ancient disease. Egyptian mummies from 4,000 years ago show signs of it, and the Greek historian Hippocrates described it as the commonest fatal disease in around 460 BCE.

Symptoms

TB is most frequently a lung disease and in this form was usually known as 'consumption' or 'phthisis', but it can also affect other parts of the

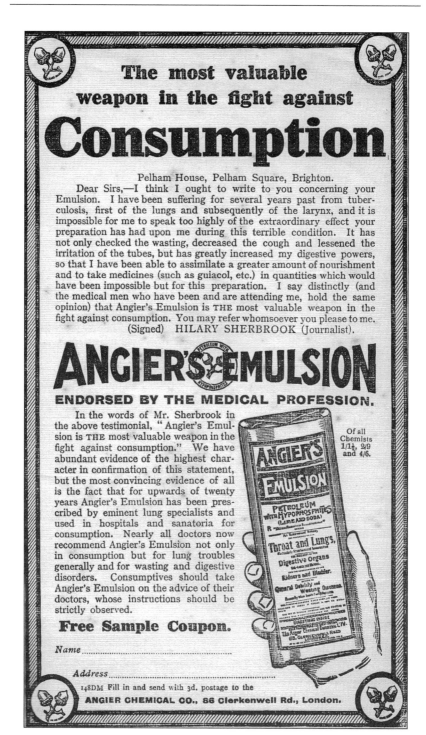

Before antibiotics, many products were promoted as cures for TB. Angier's Emulsion was advertised widely between 1890 and 1940.

body such as the skin, bones, and glands in the neck. The lung condition starts with a simple dry cough, but as the infection takes hold the cough becomes very persistent – even violent – and sufferers bring up large amounts of phlegm and sometimes blood. Patients develop fever and have a characteristically intense night-time sweating; they have little appetite, which causes weight loss, and they feel very tired. A typical TB patient with advanced disease is thin, pale, lethargic, and coughs continuously.

However, the human immune system can trap TB bacteria in thick-walled 'tubercles' in the lung where they become dormant. When this happens, patients can live a comparatively normal life afterwards. If tubercles don't isolate all the bacteria, or they rupture at some later point, the sufferer progressively weakens and eventually wastes away, often over a period of years. The disease spreads mainly because of a TB victim's coughing which broadcasts droplets of their infected sputum over others. So in crowded living conditions, TB can pass quickly from one victim to the next. The crowded urbanisation of Victorian times thus helped it to spread.

Treatments

It is hard to know if any treatment was effective for TB before the arrival of antibiotics because patients can improve spontaneously when tubercles form. Whether anything other than a balanced diet encourages this natural process is unclear, but it seems unlikely. For hundreds of years there were three staples of treatment: exercise, diet, and climate. Yet the details vary enormously with the era. For example, in the eighteenth century, vigorous exercise (e.g. horse riding) and long sea voyages were encouraged, whereas by the twentieth century, bizarre regimens of extreme rest were advocated. In the nineteenth century, fat-rich diets were all the rage, in the twentieth century cereals were popular. Physicians in all eras argued about the most suitable atmospheric conditions for their patients – cool high altitudes, warm coastal areas, or dry tropical climates?

A vast array of medicines were used. Cod liver oil was particularly popular in Victorian times. Henry Ancell in his *A Treatise on Tuberculosis* (1852) echoed the thoughts of many of his contemporary physicians: 'Cod-liver Oil: This is the most important therapeutical agent that has yet been discovered for the treatment of tuberculosis. Both children and adults who are anaemic, atrophied, and debilitated when they commence its use, become florid, active and strong, and they increase in weight.' Other Victorian treatments included iodine, quinine, and iron. A variety of highly poisonous substances were also used such as barium and mercury, and there were many brand name or 'patent' medicines.

Finding the Cause

In the 1774 edition of his book *Domestic Medicine*, the physician William Buchan reveals much about eighteenth-century thinking concerning the origins of tuberculosis – a combination of the patient's physical characteristics, diet, behaviour, and the weather:

> Consumption: Young persons, betwixt the age of fifteen and thirty, of a slender make, long neck, high shoulders, and flat breasts, are most liable to this disease. Consumptions prevail more in England than in any other part of the world, owing perhaps to the great use of animal food and malt-liquors, the general application to sedentary employments, and the great quantity of pit-coal which is there burnt; to which we may add the perpetual changes in the atmosphere, or variableness of the weather.

In nineteenth-century Britain, the medical profession vigorously scrutinised the origins of TB, believing that if they could identify the cause they would find a cure. But the basic principles of scientific investigation were not understood at this time, and so Victorian doctors gained no more insight than their eighteenth-century counterparts. Repeatedly doctors would report some chance observation in a group of TB sufferers and eagerly claim that this was the cause – or an important trigger for – the illness. A bewilderingly long list of causative factors grew and grew.

That list today seems ludicrous. As expected, Victorian values and sensibilities imposed themselves – for instance consumption of alcohol was linked to the cause of TB, as was masturbating. Some believed that TB in infants was related to the behaviour or illnesses of parents before their child's birth: for example, if the parents were of different temperaments, the mother was a lunatic, either parent had had syphilis, or the husband was too old for his wife.

Other factors linked to the development of TB included: being fair-skinned and blue-eyed, habitually adopting a bent posture, a history of depression, a deficiency of atmospheric electricity, insufficient sunlight, prolonged exposure to cold, living in unwholesome air, the taking of too many mercury and arsenic-containing medicines, adopting a sedentary lifestyle, and not washing regularly. Interestingly, some believed that TB was caused by smallpox vaccination, echoing recent mistrust about vaccine safety in our own times.

The fact that TB was so common and that sufferers needed long-term medical attention fuelled a building boom for hospitals. Before Victorian times, hospitals were few in number and often small charitable institutions, yet the new large-scale hospitals would soon be needed to meet the other health needs of a growing population quite apart from TB. Only in comparatively recent times have many of these grand old Victorian buildings been replaced by more modern facilities.

In 1882, Robert Koch swept aside the endless speculation about the origins of the disease when he discovered that TB was an infection caused by *Mycobacterium tuberculosis* – a species of bacteria. In the modern world we are so used to the concept of bacteria causing disease that it is hard for us to appreciate what a revelation this was. The *Illustrated London News* reported, with a sense of wonder, that TB was caused by 'the settlement and growth of very small animal parasites in the lungs' and that 'bacteria, as they are called, reside in infected water, some in the air, and some in living organic bodies'.

Significant progress was also made when the medical value of X-rays was pioneered in the 1890s. This allowed doctors to see inside patients' lungs and make a definitive diagnosis of TB. Some surgical techniques were also introduced – particularly collapsing one infected lung to 'rest' it.

The Twentieth Century

Unfortunately, establishing the cause and making better diagnoses did not change the outlook for victims. In fact, after all the vigorous medical attention to TB in Victorian times, it is surprising that the early twentieth century reveals a curiously lethargic approach. The mainstay of treatment by this time consisted of lying around in the fresh air all day doing nothing. Patients lay in bed at home with the windows open, in the garden, or in a specialist TB sanatorium. And woe betide that anyone – least of all the patient's family – should do anything other than strictly what the doctor ordered. One clearly exasperated doctor wrote in 1928: 'Two of the commonest contributory factors which turn the scale against or hasten the end of sufferers from pulmonary tuberculosis are over-exertion, and over-anxious, fussy, and interfering relatives.'

In 1935, *The Practical Home Doctor*, by a Harley Street Specialist, a popular home handbook on health, summarised the cutting edge of TB management of the time – staying in bed all day with the windows open:

When a person is found actually to have consumption he should first of all be put to bed and kept there for from four to six weeks at least, in order to give him complete rest. If the temperature does not fall to normal in a week or two, 'absolute rest' must be insisted upon, the patient not being allowed to feed himself or wash or get out of bed or even to read during this period. The windows of the bedroom should be kept open day and night, no matter what the weather is.

There is little doubt that the best place to treat tuberculosis is in a sanatorium, where the discipline and example of other patients is helpful.

A vaccine to prevent TB was first used in humans in 1921. BCG vaccine was a weakened strain of *Mycobacterium* that did not cause TB and was named after its two inventors: 'Bacillus Calmette Guerin'. However, the vaccine was not widely used until the 1940s, and British schoolchildren were not routinely immunised until 1953.

So, doctors now knew what caused TB, and could diagnose and prevent it. What they still couldn't do was treat it effectively.

Then in 1943 two antibiotics for TB were discovered at the same time: streptomycin and para-aminosalicylic acid. They were effective initially, but the bacteria quickly became resistant to them. However, when

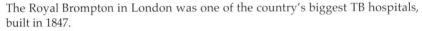

The Royal Brompton in London was one of the country's biggest TB hospitals, built in 1847.

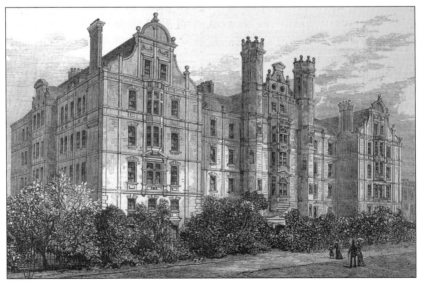

another drug, isoniazid, was introduced in 1952, scientists discovered that using the three drugs together prevented resistance. Nowadays, TB is always treated with combinations of antibiotics for the same reason, yet the number of modern antibiotics that will treat TB is extremely limited so an increasing number of cases resistant to all antibiotics are being encountered. This is a major reason behind modern media stories about a resurgence of TB, although it is on nothing like the scale that existed in the pre-antibiotic era.

Your Ancestors and Tuberculosis

Old names for tuberculosis which may be found on death certificates or in historical documents include:

- Consumption.
- Koch's disease.
- Phthisis or phthisis pulmonalis.
- Tissick.
- White plague.
- Tubercular meningitis (TB of the brain).
- King's evil or scrofula (TB of glands in neck).
- Tabes mesenterica (abdominal TB).
- Lupus vulgaris (skin TB).
- Pott's disease (bone TB).

TB was associated with persons from the lower socio-economic groups because they were more likely to live in the crowded conditions which favoured its spread. If your ancestor suffered from TB and was from a slightly wealthier background, the diagnosis may explain their sudden move to a different part of the country where the air was considered more conducive to recovery. This can show up in census returns, and may involve the family splitting up: the affected individual relocating alone leaving the rest of the family behind, or their move accompanied by only a small retinue. The fresh air of the pretty seaside town of Torquay in Devon, for example, attracted many TB sufferers to rehabilitate in the Victorian and Edwardian eras.

A number of famous British people suffered from TB including Robert Louis Stevenson, HG Wells, Vivien Leigh, Alexander Graham Bell, Sir Noël Coward, and Anne, Charlotte and Emily Brontë.

Chapter 23

TYPHUS

Typhus is an all-but-forgotten disease in the Western world, but in the past it was a common cause of our ancestors' deaths. Despite its similar name, it is a completely different illness to typhoid (see Chapter 10). Typhus occurred in densely packed communities where personal contact could happen easily, and it affected a broad spectrum of people in this situation. However, it has tended to be associated with those in the lower socio-economic groups such as prisoners, soldiers, sailors, and the crowded urban poor.

Symptoms

The initial symptoms of typhus were described well by naval surgeon Robert Robertson in *Observations on the Jail, Hospital, or Ship Fever*, 1783:

> The diagnostic symptoms, or those which generally introduce the fever, are rigors or chilliness, or alternate chills and heats; sickness at stomach, headache, universal pains (or as the sick express it: 'pains all over them') or pains in all their bones but especially in the loins or back, and a morbid appearance in the countenance.

These initial symptoms persisted throughout the illness, with the multiple sites of pain and tenderness being very distressing. The high fever that followed these first symptoms was particularly dramatic: patients became very hot indeed. They sweated profusely and became thirsty, shivery, and hoarse-voiced; at times the fever was high enough to even cause fitting. Some patients developed a relentless cough, or pains in the eyes when exposed to daylight ('photophobia'). Others had painful muscle cramps.

A characteristic feature of typhus was the 'petechiae', or small red spots on the skin that initially looked like flea bites. The spots were small

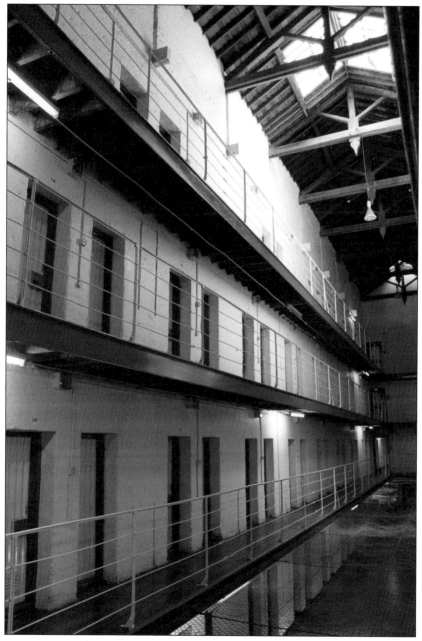

Many people were crammed into old-style prisons and this encouraged the easy spread of typhus.

and perhaps easily overlooked, but they led to typhus being known as 'petechial fever' or 'spotted fever' (although in modern medical terminology, 'spotted fever' is a distinct group of specific forms of typhus).

Some patients began to improve after a few days and recovered completely, whilst for others the symptoms gradually deteriorated. It is not clear what proportion of infected people died, but the mortality rate from contemporary accounts seems high. A log of cases at the London Fever Hospital in 1868 suggested a mortality rate of about one in seven, but other accounts can suggest much higher death rates (for example, see Pringle's account, on p. 181).

Contemporary doctors were often impressed by the longevity of illness before the patient died – sometimes extending to a fortnight. When the end came, dehydration often brought about delirium with the restless, excitable patient babbling nonsense or behaving rather inappropriately. This was followed by a lapse into semi-consciousness or stupor, and then death.

Doctors treated typhus unimaginatively with the usual bloodletting, emetics, and cathartics, plus various traditional remedies for fever such as quinine. All of these would have been ineffective.

London physician Charles Murchison described a case in his *A Treatise on the Continued Fevers of Great Britain*, 1862:

> Thomas M., aged 36, admitted into the London Fever Hospital, May 12th, 1862. Out of employment for many weeks. Was taken ill six days before admission with rigors [cold chills] and loss of appetite. Although he felt very weak, he continued going about until May 11th.
>
> On admission, pulse 96 and weak. Tongue dry and brown along the centre; bowels open from medicine. A well-marked typhus eruption [rash], the spots persistent on pressure, on chest and abdomen. Eyes injected; face flushed; answers correctly, but is rather excited; and says he is afraid to go to sleep for fear of something happening to him. Has had much pain in limbs, and headache, but the pains have almost ceased.
>
> Was ordered beef-tea and milk, four ounces of wine, and a mixture containing sulphuric acid, sulphuric ether, and quinine.
>
> April 14th (ninth day). Is more prostrate. Hands and tongue tremulous. Is stupid and confused, and occasionally delirious. Pulse 120. Tongue dry and brown. Urine passed in bed.
>
> Four ounces of brandy were ordered.

On the evening of the 14th, he had a slight convulsive fit, with foaming at the mouth, lasting for a quarter of an hour. After this he became drowsy and unconscious, and scarcely took notice when spoken to; the tremors increased and there was also subsultus [twitching]; the abdomen was tympanic [tight, like drum], and the motions and urine were passed involuntarily. The urine was ascertained to contain a considerable quantity of albumen [a protein; this means he had kidney damage].

The brandy was increased to ten ounces. A strong infusion of coffee was ordered to be taken every four hours. The bowels were freely moved and sinapisms [mustard plasters] were applied to the loins.

The patient, however, became weaker; on the 17th he was comatose and he remained in this state until his death on the 18th (thirteenth day).

Origins

Typhus was a feverish illnesses that doctors realised could move from person to person. As with many similar contagious illnesses in the era before bacteria were discovered, doctors typically blamed 'bad air' for the problem. This did, however, often encourage them to isolate patients when they could, which was a beneficial tactic as it limited the spread of the disease.

Typhus is actually an infection that is spread by human lice, which can carry bacteria called *Rickettsia*. It is the bacteria that cause typhus: the lice bite their human hosts and inadvertently inject them with *Rickettsia*. This explains the link between typhus and people living in close community with each other – physical touch enables the infection-carrying lice to move from one person to another.

James Lind – more famous for his proof that citrus fruits cured scurvy (Chapter 19) – was the first to suggest that typhus probably spread via contaminated textiles such as blankets and clothing. We now know that these materials could harbour the lice. Lind successfully reduced infection rates by keeping the hospital environment clean and by baking the clothes of new naval recruits to cleanse them. This heating would have killed the lice. Unfortunately, as with scurvy, Lind's evidence was far ahead of its time and was not widely accepted into practice.

The connection between bacteria, lice and typhus was not made until the early twentieth century. This knowledge facilitated the use of insecticides to kill the lice and prevent infection, and once antibiotics came into being they could be successfully employed to treat established typhus.

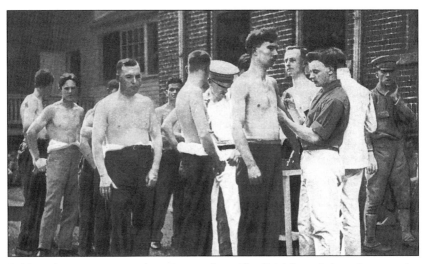

Soldiers being immunised against typhus. The British and American armies experimented with typhus vaccines in the early twentieth century – one recipient wrote to his nephew on the back of this postcard: 'Here is how they jagged our arms when they inoculated us. I bet you would faint – how about it?'

Effects of Disease

Since the disease is spread by lice, there is a limited capacity for wide-scale spread of the disease. Hence typhus has tended not to cause nationwide epidemics, but to cause intense localised outbreaks of infection within certain populations. It has been particularly associated with communities where people were forced into overly close proximity to one another such as occurs in prisons, hospitals, barracks, and on board ships. Typhus has, accordingly, earned a variety of names such as gaol fever or distemper, hospital fever, army or camp fever, and ship's fever amongst others. It was also sometimes known as 'putrid fever'.

Typhus was also commonly linked with events that brought people together en masse, such as wars, and it featured prominently as a cause of death in the English Civil War, for example, as well as in the Crimea, the trenches of the First World War, and the concentration and prisoner-of-war camps of the Second World War. It has also been closely associated with the long history of famines in Britain and especially in Ireland (see Chapter 9).

The so-called Black Assizes in England offer remarkable examples of the effects of typhus. These were criminal proceedings where prisoners became infected with typhus whilst waiting for trial. In a short space of time much of the court became infected and prisoners, witnesses, juries, barristers, and judges all succumbed. The classic series of trials referred to as Black Assizes are those in Cambridge (1522), Oxford (1577), Exeter (1586), Taunton (1730), Launceston (1742), and the Old Bailey (1750). A near contemporary account of the last of these was written by John Pringle, Physician-General to the Army in his *Observations on the Diseases of the Army*, 1753:

> The prisoners were the whole day crowded together till they were brought out to be tried: and, it appeared afterwards, that these places had not been cleaned for some years. The poisonous quality of the air was still aggravated by the heat and closeness of the court, and by the perspirable matter of a great number of all sorts of people, penned up for most part of the day, without breathing the free air, or receiving any refreshment. The bench consisted of six persons, whereof four died [including the Lord Mayor of London], together with two or three of the counsel, one of the under-sheriffs, several of the Middlesex jury, and others present, the amount of above forty in the whole; without making allowance for those of a lower rank, whose death may not have been heard of, or including any that did not sicken within a fortnight after the sessions.
>
> It was said that the fever in the beginning had an inflammatory appearance, but that after large evacuations the pulse sunk, and was not to be raised by blisters or cordials, and that the patients soon became delirious. Several had the petechiae; and all that were seized with the fever died, excepting two or three at most.

Your Ancestors and Typhus

The symptoms of typhus are not very specific and it is one of a number of illnesses that may be the cause of the 'fever' often documented in older records for the death of an ancestor. This is because physicians were often not in attendance when a person died and so were unable to make a diagnosis, but even when a doctor was present the discriminating power of professional diagnosis in former times was not great. Indeed, in the past, doctors argued over the differences between typhus and typhoid.

An adult ancestor who died of 'fever' or 'pestilential fever' may have died from typhus, and this is a reasonable working theory in a close-knit community in the absence of evidence to the contrary. The main competing diagnosis is often typhoid, since both conditions feature fever as a symptom and both spread quickly when people are in close proximity. Typhoid, being a bowel infection, causes diarrhoea but typhus does not. Other potential diagnoses for 'fever' include yellow fever and malaria, but in the last few centuries these are confined to fairly specific geographical areas (Chapter 21). Diseases such as dysentery, cholera, and scurvy occur in similar communities to typhus but do not generally cause a high body temperature so are less likely to be termed 'fever'. Influenza causes fever but operates as an epidemic or pandemic over much wider population areas than typhus.

Fever or typhus is often recorded as a cause of death in Royal Navy records such as surgeons' logs, and on crew lists and logs in the merchant navy. Records of prisons, military campaigns, and asylums may also yield evidence of the disease. Old naval ships were sometimes used as prisons in the eighteenth and nineteenth centuries, and their records may reveal an ancestor's fate. For example, an inquest was held on board the prison ship HMS *Racoon* at Portsmouth Harbour on 3 June 1825, upon the body of Thomas Hills. He was a convict, and the proceedings concluded that he died of typhus fever (reference HCA 1/105 at TNA).

As with dysentery, the close confines of a ship could enable typhus infection to spread quickly to devastating effect. Emigrant ships in the nineteenth century were particularly susceptible to typhus because the passengers were packed together so tightly. The *Quebec Chronicle* for 1847 records these mortality rates on emigrant ships arriving in Canada in that year:

Vessels	Where From	Passengers on Board	Died of Ship Fever
Goliah	Liverpool	600	46
Charles Richards	Sligo	178	8
Medusa	Cork	194	2
Alert	Waterford	234	4
Jordine	Liverpool	354	8
Manchester	Liverpool	512	11
Jessie	Cork	437	37
Erin's Queen	Liverpool	517	50
Sarah	Liverpool	248	31
Rosana	Cork	254	3
Triton	Liverpool	483	90
Thistle	Liverpool	389	8
Avon	Cork	550	136
		Total = 4,950	Total = 434

Chapter 24

VENEREAL DISEASES

The term 'venereal disease' is derived from Venus, the Roman goddess of love, and was widely used until the mid-twentieth century to refer to any sexually transmitted disease.

It is generally believed that syphilis was introduced to the rest of the world from the Americas because it was unknown in Europe until the mid-1490s when Columbus's crew returned from their epic trans-Atlantic crossing. Indeed, Christopher Columbus himself is believed to have suffered from the disease which was known as the Great Pox (to distinguish it from smallpox). Reaching a population with no natural immunity, syphilis spread rapidly and in a form that seems a lot more severe than the modern disease: patients reported large stinking pustules, debilitating ulcers which quickly ate down to the bone, and a great deal of pain. Yet by the early sixteenth century it had already been noted that patients who became infected were faring much better than in the recent past, so the disease seems to have quickly changed its character and become milder.

Gonorrhoea is a different disease that had been known in Europe long before the arrival of syphilis, but until the nineteenth century many believed the two conditions were stages of the same illness.

Symptoms
Classically, syphilis starts with an ulcer near the site of infection (a chancre) and swelling of the lymph glands (buboes). The secondary phase is characterised by fever, sore throat, bone aches, and rashes. The tertiary stage is most serious and develops years later; it includes sores and swellings throughout the body (gummata) that eat into bone, internal organs and the face, and can cause gross disfigurement. It can also cause brain damage resulting in a range of psychiatric and neurological problems such as dementia, psychosis, convulsions, and muscle weakness; this was often called 'general paralysis of the insane' in the nineteenth century.

The main features of gonorrhoea are a discharge from the genitals, pain on urinating, and tenderness in the groin area.

Attitudes to VD

Being a particularly unpleasant disease, the English naturally named syphilis after their nearest Continental rival, from whence they assumed it came, and it became widely known as the 'French Pox'. Throughout the world there was a cascade of similar xenophobic labelling – the French called it the 'Disease of Naples', to the Turks it was the 'Christian Disease', the Japanese identified it as the 'Portuguese Sickness', and so forth.

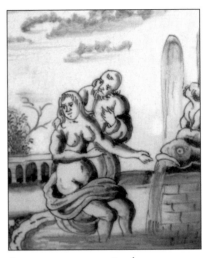

An amorous encounter for our ancestors risked infection with venereal disease.

Society didn't just blame nasty foreigners for venereal diseases, there was an element of divine retribution as well. VD was perceived as an illness that marked the sufferer as unclean both physically and morally. It was particularly associated with prostitution, dirtiness, and indulging in excesses of all kinds. The Christian church's view was that sexual intercourse was a means for creating children with a single marriage partner, and was not a pleasure to be indulged in wantonly – so VD was seen by some as God's punishment for dissolute behaviour. Despite this, the Vatican established St Fiacre as the patron saint of VD sufferers. (Somewhat incongruously he is also the patron saint of haemorrhoid sufferers and taxi drivers.)

Male-dominated societies identified promiscuous women as responsible for the spread of VD – especially prostitutes – who 'harboured' the disease ready to infect unsuspecting men. So, for example, when the first purpose-built British hospital for venereal disease was founded in 1746 it initially dealt only with female patients: the London Lock Hospital was established near Hyde Park. It developed a rescue home providing accommodation and domestic training for some ex-patients. In 1862 a separate site was developed for male patients. It wasn't until 1867 that a survey showed that 36 per cent of women admitted to the hospital were 'married women infected with venereal disease by their husbands, or in a manner wholly devoid of blame to themselves'.

The Victorians' prudishness about all matters sexual prevented anyone publicly identifying the real extent of the problem or warning the population about the dangers of unsafe sex. The diagnosis of VD was considered highly shameful and the desire to hide the condition led victims to spread the infection amongst their sexual contacts.

Incidence

Some rather alarming figures suggest that VD was surprisingly common in Victorian society. For instance, army records show that amongst 73,000 British personnel there were a staggering 20,600 hospitalisations for VD in 1865. Furthermore, London doctors in 1868 estimated that between one-fifth and one-third of all patients attending hospital for any reason were suffering from VD. For some hospitals it was even worse – Guy's Hospital reported that 43 per cent of their outpatients were suffering from VD, and 50 per cent of all surgical patients at St Bartholomew's were infected.

The government decided that tackling the prostitutes would stem the tide of infection. The Contagious Diseases Act of 1864 regulated prostitution in certain areas of the country – particularly near army bases or ports. Prostitutes were regularly arrested and examined for VD; those found to be infected were forcibly detained in hospital until cured, which could take up to a year. There was no legal sanction to examine or force treatment upon male clients and this made it controversial, even at the time. The Act may have had some localised success – for example, Plymouth naval base reported 13 per cent of men with VD in 1864, but only 5 per cent in 1867. Nonetheless, the Act proved impossible to police in practice, and unpopular, and it was repealed in 1886.

Venereal disease has always been a particular concern for the armed forces. As early as the eighteenth century the navy tried to identify and treat sufferers and they are often named in surgeons' logs or paybooks. However, infection rates in all services continued to increase into the twentieth century: during the First World War, for example, there were over 400,000 hospital admissions for venereal diseases amongst British military personnel. It wasn't until late in the Second World War that the government finally launched any kind of health promotion concerning VD in Britain and this was aimed at servicemen. Their posters still effectively branded women as the cause of the problem.

One anonymous Second World War navy rating recalled his encounter with the disease in 1945.

I went to see the MO [medical officer] because I had this pain when I peed. Before he even examined me, he went straight into a talk about the dangers of 'the clap' and how we boys ought to be more careful: I had the full works about sex, prostitutes, condoms ... everything.

I was only 17 and got embarrassed. Those things weren't talked about where I came from. There was no privacy and the men outside probably heard everything. I said I must have caught it from a toilet seat or something.

'Young man' he said sternly 'only the chaplain and officers above the rank of commander are *allowed* to catch VD from a toilet seat'.

Congenital Syphilis

Untreated syphilis in a woman can seriously affect the outcome of any pregnancies, causing miscarriage, premature delivery, stillbirth, or the death of the baby shortly after delivery. Babies that survive are often of low birth weight and may show signs of being infected with the syphilis that their mother has passed onto them in the womb. This is called congenital or constitutional syphilis. Early signs of the baby's infection may be seen within three months of being born such as serious kidney or bone damage, rashes, and meningitis. Late signs of congenital syphilis come on once the child is over 2 years of age and can include progressive blindness, atypical facial features, swollen joints, and mental retardation. These children may also suddenly become deaf – often at around 8 to 10 years of age. Fits and symptoms of mental illness may result if syphilis enters the infant's brain.

The rate of transmission of syphilis from mother to baby is affected by the time that has elapsed since the woman was originally infected. Kassowitz's law states that the greater the interval between mother being infected and her becoming pregnant, then the better outcome there is likely to be for the baby.

In practical terms this means that a recently infected woman is more likely to experience miscarriages for her first few pregnancies. Subsequent pregnancies may result in stillbirths and then babies who die young. Pregnancies that follow on after this may produce babies that survive but who are unwell due to congenital syphilis, until after several years there is a return to near-normal health with babies being born in good physical shape. This pattern may sometimes come to light when researching your family tree.

Treatments

From the sixteenth century, various American plants were advocated to treat VD. Guaiacum or 'holy' wood was particularly popular for syphilis, but others included sarsaparilla and cinchona. For gonorrhoea, physicians usually advocated light diet, laxatives, avoidance of strong-flavoured foods, and the injection of oils, zinc solutions, and other substances into the genitals.

However, by far the most enduring treatment for syphilis or gonorrhoea was mercury which was applied to affected sores as an ointment, used as a solution to irrigate the genitals, inhaled as a vapour, or taken by mouth as pills. A very popular form of mercury was calomel (or mercurous chloride), another was known as the 'blue pill'. Unfortunately, mercury is extremely toxic, especially if taken long-term, and users commonly reported signs of poisoning such as profuse sweating, skin damage, loose teeth, mood swings, and kidney failure. How effective it really was is unclear, yet from the seventeenth century its fame was such that this saying became well known: 'A night in the arms of Venus leads to a life on mercury'.

The physician William Buchan described his general approach to treatment of venereal diseases in the 1790 edition of his book *Domestic Medicine*:

> Although it is impossible, on account of the different degrees of virulence etc, to lay down fixed and certain rules for the cure of this disease, yet the following general plan will always be found safe, and often successful, *viz* to bleed the patient and administer gentle purges with diuretics during the initial inflammatory state, and as soon as the symptoms of inflammation are abated, to administer mercury, in any form that may be most agreeable to the patient. The same medicine, assisted by the decoction of sarsaparilla, and a proper regimen, will not only secure the constitution against the further progress of a confirmed pox, but will generally perform a complete cure.

A whole series of branded medicines were promoted as VD cures from the eighteenth to the early twentieth centuries including Clarke's Blood Mixture, Santal de Midy solution, Leake's Pills, and Kennedy's Lisbon Diet Drink. Some products, such as Hannay's Preventive, claimed to protect against infection.

The bacterial origin of gonorrhoea, *Neisseria gonorrhoeae*, was described by Albert Neisser in 1879 and that for syphilis, *Treponema pallidum*, by

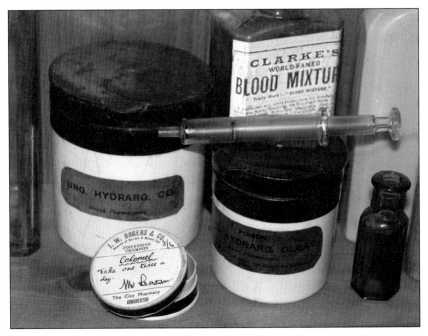

Late nineteenth and early twentieth-century medicines for venereal disease.

Schaudinn and Hoffmann in 1905. Once the cause was known, science was on a surer footing when hunting for a cure.

The first specific treatment for syphilis was an arsenic compound known as Salvarsan, launched in 1910 but it had to be injected, required long-term treatment and could cause serious side effects. The first treatment for gonorrhoea came with sulphonamide antibiotics in 1937 but the bacteria became resistant to them very quickly. So, it was not until penicillin tablets were introduced in 1943 that there was an effective, safe, and quick treatment for VD.

Your Ancestors and VD

Syphilis and gonorrhoea were known as 'social diseases', Cupid's disease, the curse of Venus, or 'the clap', the latter term being used mainly (but not exclusively) for gonorrhoea.

Perhaps surprisingly, there are archive resources where you can still identify ancestors who were diagnosed with VD. Royal Navy records can be a source of such information. The eighteenth and nineteenth-century musters or paybooks from Royal Navy ships at TNA sometimes include lists of men who were treated by a visiting pox doctor. For example, the records of HMS *Greyhound* declare: 'Received the 2nd August 1781, nineteen pounds and ten shillings for the venereal cures performed by Mr James Ballyntine and charged hereon'. The accompanying 'venereal list' identifies eleven culprits who were administered Mr Ballyntine's dubious cures including John Holmes, Simon Allen, and John Swiney. Other sources include service records, and the official logs kept by naval surgeons.

Records from some hospitals that specialised in treating VD have also survived. For example, records relating to the London Lock Hospital for 1746 to 1948 are held by the Royal College of Surgeons (series MS 0022), and include some patient records dating back as far as the eighteenth century. Access to this collection is via written application to The Archivist, Royal College of Surgeons of England, 35–43 Lincoln Inn Fields, London WC2A 3PN.

If your ancestor suffered from VD, then you may take heart from the fact that many well-known figures from history suffered, or are believed to have suffered, from VD. They include Adolf Hitler, Napoleon Bonaparte, Henry VIII, Oscar Wilde, Franz Schubert, Al Capone, Edouard Manet, Pope Alexander VI, and Ivan the Terrible.

Chapter 25

WAR

Armed conflict means that people die – but civilians are killed as well as military professionals, and wars can have a legacy of death that extends beyond the period of fighting. This is illustrated well by the merciless progress of the parliamentary forces in the Civil War, as shown in this account that was reproduced in *The True Briton*, 1752:

> And in this year 1649, there was a famine in Lancashire and the northern counties occasioned by the frequent ravages, marches, and spoil of the soldiers. And when Cromwell took Drogheda in Ireland, he put the whole garrison to the sword, consisting of about 3,000 men, most English, insomuch that only one lieutenant escaped; he also murdered every man, woman, and child of the citizens that were Irish.

The death toll from armed conflict has escalated as the centuries have ticked by. The Commonwealth War Graves Commission, for example, cares for memorials dedicated to around 1.7 million British military and merchant navy personnel who died in the two world wars – including from Empire and Commonwealth countries. This organisation has also recorded the deaths of around 67,000 British civilians in the Second World War.

Military Personnel
In wartime, those who do the fighting are clearly at high risk of being killed by the enemy. It is an awful reflection of the large numbers of men killed in the two world wars that many were reported 'missing presumed dead' because no body was ever found. This is particularly true of deaths at sea, and in the trenches of the First World War. Yet the enemy can kill military personnel other than in the heat of the conflict – you may find an ancestor who was detained during hostilities and then shot trying to

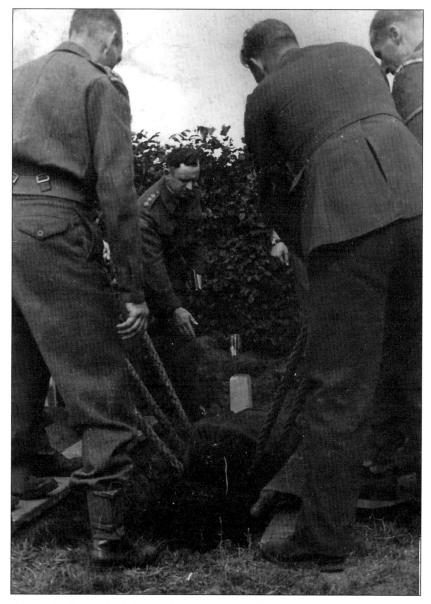

Soldiers in the First World War burying a comrade.

escape imprisonment, who was executed for a wartime offence, or who died due to the unhealthy conditions in a prisoner-of-war camp.

Notwithstanding these deaths caused directly by the enemy's forces, disease has been a prominent feature of many wars. Massing a large body of men together in one place in a camp or a fleet can encourage the rapid spread of infection and strain the ability of even the best commanders to maintain the health of their men. Thus typhus outbreaks amongst the armies of the English Civil War were notorious; scurvy killed more eighteenth-century Royal Navy seamen than the French; and the loss of soldiers in the Crimea due to diseases such as cholera and dysentery scandalised Victorian society. These diseases are all the subject of other chapters in this book.

Trench fever was a significant problem in the First World War. We now know that it was spread by a species of bacteria (*Bartonella quintana*) carried by human lice, but this was only partially understood during the conflict. The following account is taken from the *Cleveland Medical Journal*, 1918:

> Trench fever is a real war problem. The real cause is not known, but it seems to be caused by some specific organism that is transmitted by the body louse or 'cootie'. The knowledge of its transmission allows only a partial protection, however, and its prevention really depends on knowing the inciting organism. Much work is being done on this, especially by the English, and on two occasions it was thought that the organism was isolated but the work has since been shown to be erroneous. Control of the disease would be a very great help, as 20 per cent of the 'sick' cases are trench fever.

Symptoms included a fever that broke out in cycles every five days or so, weakness, lethargy, muscle pains, painful shins, headache, a rash, and a sore abdomen. Although trench fever rarely killed soldiers directly, it weakened those who were infected so that they might be disabled from fighting for months. This could render them more susceptible to other disease, whilst those who did not leave the front line in time, or who returned too soon, were less 'fighting fit' and so probably more at risk from dying in battle.

The disease known as 'trench foot' was another major health concern in the First World War, and was caused by soldiers standing around in water-filled trenches for days at a time. The unrelenting coldness cut off the circulation and the perpetual exposure to water softened the skin so that it broke down more easily. These effects together caused infections and sores, which could ultimately lead to gangrene and then amputation (see Chapter 26).

The First World War also witnessed a novel and terrible weapon. Not an innovative bullet, blade, or explosive, but a drifting airborne killer –

gas. The principal substances used for this new chemical warfare were chlorine, phosgene, and mustard gas, but a variety of other agents were employed, each with different properties. Many of these chemicals damaged the lungs and could lead to a lingering death as victims effectively drowned in the fluids that their own inflamed lungs produced. Men that survived serious gas exposure suffered from 'weak chests' for the rest of their lives, which limited their activity and predisposed them to chest infections. Certain gases could also cause blindness and skin blistering.

Yet disease and the enemy's weapons were not the only mortal dangers faced by someone fighting for their country. A member of the armed forces might be killed by someone fighting on his or her own side. Courts martial could be ordered for a variety of offences including, most notably, desertion. For example, in 1797, whilst Britain was at war with France,

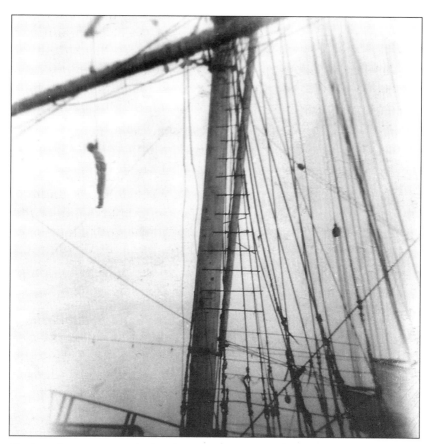

The Royal Navy only abolished hanging from the yardarm in 1860.

the Royal Navy caught up with able seaman Joseph Prout at Halifax, after he had deserted HMS *Assistance*. He was given 200 lashes which was in effect the very cruel sentence of being flogged to death. Mutineers were traditionally hanged from the yardarm in the navy. During the First World War, the British army executed 346 of its own men – usually for desertion, but also for cowardice, or failure to follow orders. These desperate individuals, with whom many of us can empathise, faced a firing squad. They are listed on the Shot at Dawn website at www.shotatdawn.info.

Finally, many fighting personnel who survived a conflict found that they suffered because of it, emotionally or physically, for many years afterwards. In some cases intractable pain or the effects of field surgery, and problems such as mental illness or alcoholism – resulting from the sights, experiences, and consequences of war – led to a sad death many years after the conflict, sometimes self-inflicted. There is heart-rending footage of young soldiers suffering some of the physical manifestations of shell shock from the First World War on the Wellcome Library website at http://catalogue.wellcome.ac.uk/record=b1667864~S8.

Civilians

Britain has been spared the costs of large-scale, land-based conflict on its own soil since the Battle of Culloden in 1746, but before then many of our non-combatant ancestors became unwillingly embroiled in military actions. The seventeenth century was a particularly turbulent time with numerous pitched battles: our forebears having to deal with repeated engagements in Scotland, the English Civil War, the Glorious Revolution, and the Monmouth Rebellion.

Non-combatants suffered in wars when communities were attacked, besieged, bombed, or cut off from the outside world. And civilians weren't just killed by enemy soldiers, they were starved, executed, raped, and exposed to disease. Often these events were linked – people weakened by lack of food, for example, could neither fight nor fend off illness so well.

Some non-fighting personnel that accompany the military machine are exposed to particular dangers such as nurses and medical personnel. Another example is Britain's merchant navy, which has been targeted by enemy forces for centuries because, as islands, the nation has depended upon trade from across the sea to bring in raw materials. Sometimes merchant ships have carried light armaments or a Royal Navy escort yet the principal means of safety has always been evading the enemy's notice where possible, and then trying to outrun them if spotted. Despite this lack of fighting capability, merchant ships and their crews have tended to be regarded as 'fair game' during wars. However, whilst before the twentieth century ships were captured by the enemy and their crews imprisoned, the advent of the world wars heralded a new era whereby merchant ships – even passenger ships – were considered as legitimate targets of war and sunk with appalling loss of life.

Twentieth-century warfare saw another new and frightening threat to civilians. The introduction of aeroplanes and rockets enabled long-distance bombing. Whilst the initial targets for this activity were mainly military ones, in which civilians were sometimes caught up, increasingly the targets became the civilians themselves. This bombing was designed to smash the infrastructure of a city and the morale of its population.

The threat to civilians might not end when hostilities ceased, because afterwards might come the victor's vengeance. The convictions meted out by Judge Jeffreys in the West Country after the Monmouth Rebellion have attained historical notoriety for the Crown's cruel revenge. The 'Bloody Assizes', as they have become known, resulted in the execution of over 300 rebels at Taunton. Similarly, in 1537, following revolts in the north of England, Henry VIII ordered over 200 executions.

Your Ancestors and War

A detailed discussion on how to trace ancestors who fought in a war, or who were affected by it, is beyond the scope of this book. However, there are books in this Pen & Sword series devoted, for example, to ancestors who served in the Royal Navy, army, Royal Marines, Royal Air Force, and merchant navy. Where newspapers survive for an era of conflict, they offer invaluable contemporary accounts of the events concerned, as well as individual obituaries, illustrations, and accounts of awards for bravery.

The Commonwealth War Graves Commission website, www.cwgc.org, enables you to trace ancestors who died in the world wars, and the Veterans UK site performs a similar task for men and women killed in later conflicts, www.veterans-uk.info. Most military records and official accounts of wars across the centuries are kept at TNA. Their website at www.nationalarchives.gov.uk has a series of very useful 'research guides' describing the records available for every military service with notes on how to use them; some records are even available to download in full without having to visit the archives in person.

Chapter 26

WOUNDS

Survival after wounding is determined by the location of the injury and its nature – deep, shallow, dirty, clean, puncture, gash. A large wound, or an injury to a critical part of the body, may kill a person outright – a bullet through the head, a deep stab wound to the chest and so forth. If the function of a vital organ such as the heart is compromised, or the person loses enough blood, they will die. Yet people can die from even comparatively minor wounds if infection takes hold.

In the modern world we know that it's important to keep a wound clean to prevent infection. This has become such an established part of medical self-care that we do it without really thinking about it. But until the late nineteenth century, our ancestors had no understanding of bacteria or 'germs' because they had not been discovered. Indeed, guided by ancient physicians, such as the second-century Galen, many doctors believed that one of the clearest signs of infection – pus – was an essential feature of the healthy healing of a wound. It was sometimes called 'laudable pus' in medieval times and, disastrously, clean wounds without pus might even be deliberately contaminated in order to provoke its appearance.

But not all cultures, and not all physicians and surgeons, believed that pus was essential to healing. Even in ancient times some practitioners believed in practices that empirically seemed to produce better healing, such as washing wounds with wine, or using pitch to seal the severed end of a limb following amputation. Similarly, after a flogging in the navy, men's bloody wounds were usually cleansed with saltwater or vinegar. We now know that all these practices had an antiseptic effect.

Despite a lack of understanding of the need to keep wounds sterile it is remarkable that many of our ancestors survived horrific injuries. The practice of drilling a hole in the skull (or 'trepanning') to treat brain disorders was an established practice until the early medieval period, and archaeological evidence shows that many patients survived because the bone around the hole began to grow back. Wars often produced the most horrendous wounds, but we know of many impossible-sounding survivals before the era of sterile surgery including, most famously perhaps, the amputation of Nelson's right arm.

However, the real value of a sterile approach to wound care did not begin to be understood until the late nineteenth century, and it started with surgery. Joseph Lister, the pioneer of antiseptic surgery, reviewed published scientific work and concluded that it would be beneficial to employ chemical solutions to clean surgical instruments before using them. He found that infection rates were reduced if surgeons washed their hands, the operating table, and their instruments with carbolic acid before surgery, and he wrote about this in the *British Medical Journal*, 1867:

> Since the antiseptic treatment has been brought into full operation, and wounds and abscesses no longer poison the atmosphere with putrid exhalations, my wards, though in other respects under precisely the same circumstances as before, have completely changed their character; so that during the last nine months not a single instance of pyaemia [sepsis], hospital gangrene, or erysipelas [a skin infection] has occurred in them.

Lister also employed dressings soaked in carbolic acid and noticed far superior results during healing.

An operating theatre in about 1900 – primitive compared to today.

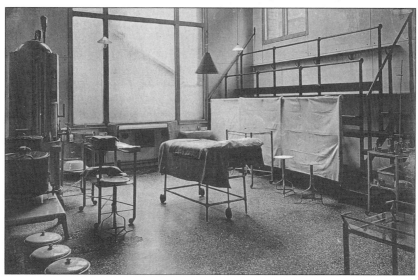

The infections that might arise from a wound can take many forms. Local infection might make a wound hot, inflamed, swollen, and filled with pus. In former times, the production of pus was called 'suppuration' and the deterioration of the wound and surrounding tissues was termed 'corruption' or 'putrefaction'. Local infections sometimes resolve by themselves, thanks to the human body's own defences, but infected material might also be cut out by a surgeon or the wound incised to release the pus. Randle Holme, a seventeenth-century surgeon, described how hooked instruments called 'drawers' were used to 'scrape out corruption in a wound or bruise'. Rather horrible in an era without anaesthesia, but necessary.

Surface wounds might also turn into ulcers – long-standing wounds that refused to heal and were often painful – particularly in older persons. Yet there were three particular consequences of an infected wound that might prove rapidly fatal: gangrene, sepsis, and tetanus.

Gangrene and Amputation

When human tissues are heavily damaged, the integrity of veins and arteries are disrupted so that the remaining flesh may not receive enough blood. This means that the body's normal bloodborne defences against infection cannot work, and bacteria begin to take hold. One species in particular can be rapidly lethal. It is called *Clostridium perfringens* and it is the main agent of gangrene. Infection with this organism means that the tissues are beginning to decompose and cannot be salvaged.

In the era before antibiotics, doctors were always aware that gangrene might supervene after any significant injury. It was initially detected by the loss of sensation in the affected part which felt cold and numb, and a change in skin colour to red and then brown and finally black. Gangrene after an injury is usually very painful. If the gangrene progressed beyond this stage, then later symptoms would include the smell of decomposing tissue, fever, and the delirium of the patient. If it reached this point then the patient inevitably died.

Gangrene was also known as 'mortification', or 'sphacelus', and was understandably much feared, especially by military men who knew it as an occupational hazard. Early amputation was the recommended treatment after any severe limb injury sustained in battle since the conditions of wartime meant that a clean wound was almost unheard-of.

Nelson's amputation has already been mentioned, but it is a good example of eighteenth-century attitudes to this practice in the military. A musket ball had shattered the bones of his forearm whilst he was trying to land a raiding party from a small boat. These days his bones might have been reconstructed, but in the eighteenth century this was impossible, and such an injury was regarded by surgeons and fighting men alike as an inevitable precursor to gangrene. As the injured Nelson stepped back on board his ship in 1797 he barked: 'Tell the surgeon to make haste and get his instruments. I know I must lose my right arm; so the sooner it is off the better.'

Surgeons knew that if the gangrenous part of the limb was not removed soon, then the affliction could spread further and overwhelm the patient. Often, as in Nelson's case, a decision was taken to amputate before any symptoms appeared because the prognosis was very much better. Amputation itself was not, of course, without risk. In the centuries before antiseptics, the operation might lead to other fatal infections, but patients might also die from shock (loss of blood or haemorrhage), and even those that survived might experience ongoing pain for years afterwards and lose their livelihoods.

Artificial limbs to replace a missing leg, arm, foot, or hand have been known for more than 2,000 years. However, until the nineteenth century these tended to be either cosmetic with no functionality, or to have only very basic functions – literally, for example, a wooden leg ('pin') or a metal hook for a hand. In the nineteenth century, simple articulating joints began to become more easily available, and were usually made of wood. In 1857, one well-known London proprietor, William Robert Grossmith, described (in his *Amputations and Artificial Limbs*, 1857) a series of the cases where he had fitted artificial limbs, including 'Miss F' who suffered an accident in 1837:

> This young lady was run over in Fleet Street, and amputated by Mr Lloyd of Bartholomew's Hospital. Being then a child she wore a common pin leg for some years till she had attained her full growth. Had my Artificial Limb in 1850, and is very expert in using it; walking, running, and dancing with perfect ease. She has never suffered the least pain or uneasiness from its use, and writes thus, March 1857: 'I should be very sorry indeed to have to use my wooden leg again even for a day. I have seen many wearing artificial legs, but none who walk as well as I do'.

The cases of Nelson and Miss F illustrates that it was possible for our ancestors who were amputees to continue in gainful employment despite a severe injury, even though the options for limb replacement were limited. When George III hinted that Nelson's injury would deprive the country of his future services, the indignant Admiral retorted that 'so

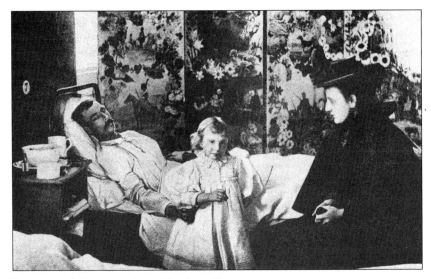

Recovery after amputation took a long time.

long as I have a foot to stand on I will combat for my King and country'. Clearly, Nelson was in a privileged position politically and financially compared to most amputees, but even those of more humble origins could sustain a living with the support of their families and local community. I noted in Chapter 3, the case of my ancestor James Wills who ran a shop, a pub, and a ship despite losing both his hands in 1842.

Sepsis

Like many medical terms, the word 'sepsis' was used more freely in the past than it is now and referred to a condition where the patient was overwhelmed by infection or 'purulence'. Sepsis was also known as septicaemia, pyaemia, suppurative fever, purulent fever, or 'blood poisoning', although some doctors argued about the definitions of these words and whether they meant precisely the same thing. From the late nineteenth century onwards, 'sepsis' could describe almost any infection that had spread from an initial focus, such a wound, to engulf the whole body via the bloodstream. For example, it was known as a problem that might manifest after major trauma or surgery and, in the era before bacteria had been discovered, Peter Braidwood described it thus in *On Pyaemia or Suppurative Fever*, 1868:

> Pyaemia may be defined to be a fever which, attacking persons
> of all ages, is generally sequent on wounds, acute inflammation

of bone, the puerperal state, surgical operations or other sources of purulent formation, and septic infection. It appears sometimes to prevail in an epidemic form. No one cause has as yet been found to produce this disease.

... The symptoms most pathognomic [characteristic] of suppurative fever are: a more or less sudden invasion on the 4th or 5th day after an operation marked generally by rigors [cold chills] or by depression of spirits and great anxiety, followed by profuse perspirations; the pulse is generally rapid; the tongue is furred, then loaded, and by and bye, brown and dry; the skin assumes a dusky sallow and then a somewhat icteric [yellow] tinge; there is very great prostration and emaciation; one or more of the joints swell, become red and painful, and may even suppurate; the breath has a heavy sweetish or purulent odour; and there is laboured respiration, delirium, or other symptoms indicative of other organs being chiefly involved.

Braidwood was not correct when he stated that sepsis might take an epidemic form, and this illustrates the confusion that existed in medical minds at the time between diseases that could cause fever.

Sepsis might arise from many other infections including scarlet fever, typhoid, maternal infections after childbirth, and skin infections such as erysipelas. Unfortunately, in the centuries before antibiotics were introduced, sepsis almost invariably killed the patient.

Tetanus

This condition arises when a particular species of bacteria, *Clostridium tetani*, enters the body via a deep wound. These bacteria live in soil and in the gut of many animals, so classically the injury that causes tetanus is a puncture-type wound such as stabbing the foot with a garden fork whilst digging the garden, or a bite from an animal. For example, Colonel George Montagu was an English naturalist who died of tetanus in 1815 after stepping on a nail sticking up from a piece of wood. However, outside the domestic setting, tetanus could also be the result of a penetrating wound experienced in time of war since such wounds were never sterile. As one First World War doctor noted, 'here, every wound is an infected one'. Whatever the circumstances of the injury, the key fact is that tetanus or 'lockjaw' only occurred after sustaining a dirty, deep wound.

Physician, Henry Clutterbuck, gave a good description of the clinical appearance of tetanus in the early nineteenth century in his 'Lectures on the diseases of the nervous system', the *Lancet*, 1826:

The first symptom of tetanus usually perceived is a degree of stiffness or rigidity of the muscles of the jaw, making it difficult either to open or shut the mouth; the mouth generally remaining nearly but not quite closed. Hence the term 'locked jaw' (trismus). By degrees the stiffness or rigidity extends to the muscles of the neck, and subsequently to those of the trunk and extremities, till the affection becomes universal. The body and limbs are rigid and inflexible, and the muscles, from the state of contraction they are in, feel as hard as a board almost …

The contraction of muscles in tetanus, though constant, is not equal or uniform, but is increased from time to time, and is then attended with increase of suffering to the patient. The disease comes on gradually, getting worse from day to day, and becoming more violent and extensive …

In a great proportion of cases the disease proves fatal; the pulse becomes quicker and smaller, and general convulsions take place before death.

Tetanus cannot be transmitted from one person to another – it is not contagious – so it affects only the individual with the wound contaminated with *Clostridium* bacteria. Nowadays all children and young adults are vaccinated against tetanus to prevent the distressingly painful death that many of our ancestors had to endure.

Chapter 27

PLACES TO VISIT

There are a number of places that you might visit which have a particular association with the deaths of our ancestors or their medical experiences.

Cemeteries and Memorials

Churches, churchyards and cathedrals across Britain are good places to see memorials to those who have died. However, there are many civic cemeteries in the country that are notable attractions. Some large ones have societies that support and care for them and in many cases their websites give details of famous incumbents, provide indexes of memorial inscriptions, or even advertise guided walks. Examples include:

Angus Kirkyards – the historic churchyards of Angus in Scotland are part of a heritage trail; www.angusheritage.com/Places/Kirkyards/Places-Kirkyards.aspx.

Belfast Cemeteries – there are many cemeteries in Belfast, including Shankhill which is over a thousand years old. Those which are now closed may be visited by appointment; www.belfastcity.gov.uk/cemeteries.

Brookwood Cemetery, Surrey – the biggest cemetery in Britain, and originally housed the excess of deceased persons that London could not accommodate; www.tbcs.org.uk.

Bunhill Fields, London – this large burial ground for Nonconformists in London's Islington, includes the grave of Daniel Defoe; www.cityoflondon.gov.uk/things-to-do/green-spaces/city-gardens;

Cathays Cemetery, Cardiff – Britain's third largest cemetery covering over 100 acres; www.rootsweb.ancestry.com/~wlsfcc/Cathays.htm.

Cholera cemeteries – many communities set aside separate burial grounds for cholera victims in the nineteenth century. Examples include:

- Belfast Cholera Cemetery, Stranmillis Road, Belfast BT9 5FE (appointment only).
- Cefn Golau Cholera Cemetery, near Tredegar, Gwent, Wales.
- Cholera Burial Ground, Station Road, York YO24 (opposite Royal York Hotel).

A number of public memorials to the victims of cholera can also be found across the country, including:

- Cholera Cross, Clay Woods, near railway station, Sheffield S2.
- Cholera Memorial, St James's Park, Paisley PA3 2LB.

Glasgow Necropolis – one of the most impressive cemeteries in Britain on account of its hilltop location overlooking the city and the grandeur of its tombs; www.glasgownecropolis.org.

Greyfriars Kirkyard, Edinburgh – includes possibly the most famous pet memorial in Britain: the loyal dog Greyfriars Bobby traditionally guarded his master's grave for over a decade; www.greyfriars.org.

Highgate Cemetery, London – a very large cemetery in north London with many famous interments including Karl Marx and Michael Faraday; www.highgate-cemetery.org.

Howff Graveyard, Dundee – a large cemetery with monuments dating back to the sixteenth century; www.howffcemetery.info.

Plague Cross, Ross-on-Wye – the inhabitants of this Herefordshire town erected a large memorial known as the Plague Cross to commemorate the local people who died in the 1637 outbreak of plague who were hastily buried in mass graves.

Southampton Old Cemetery – includes memorials to many crew members of the ill-fated *Titanic*; http://fosoc.org/.

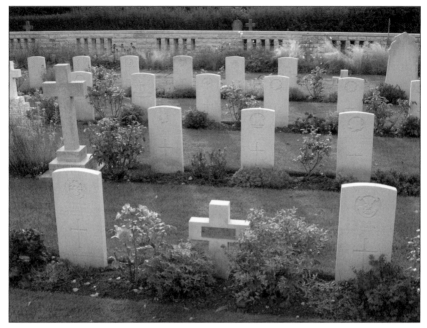

The neatly tended headstones at a Commonwealth War Graves Commission site; the Commission looks after graves and memorials from both world wars.

War Graves – the Commonwealth War Graves Commission website will help you find the last resting place or a memorial to most of the dead who fought in the world wars; www.cwgc.org.

Famous Health Professionals

Alexander Fleming Laboratory Museum, London – see the reconstructed laboratory in its original location, where penicillin was discovered in 1928; www.imperial.nhs.uk/aboutus/museumsand archives.

Edward Jenner's House and Museum, Berkeley, Gloucestershire – the house where the father of immunology lived and a museum related to the history of vaccination; www.jennermuseum.com.

Florence Nightingale Museum, London – the museum in her name houses memorabilia and artefacts connected with Nightingale and nursing; www.florence-nightingale.co.uk.

John Snow – a reconstruction of the public water pump via which Dr John Snow concluded that cholera was waterborne can be found at

Broadwick Street, London W1F 9QP. Appropriately enough, it is located next to the John Snow public house.

Hospital and Health Museums

Many large museums have a collection related to the treatment of disease such as the Museum of London and the Science Museum, both in the capital, but listed below are some less well-known attractions that specialise in particular aspects of healthcare:

Anaesthesia Heritage Centre, London – learn about the history of anaesthesia from 1846 to the present day; www.aagbi.org/education/heritage-centre.

Army Medical Services Museum, Mytchett, Surrey – the history and development of army healthcare from the seventeenth century onwards; www.ams-museum.org.uk/museum.

Bethlem Royal Hospital Archives and Museum, London – Britain's first health institution to specialise in the mentally ill; www.bethlemheritage.org.uk. The website describes the archive collection of documents, exhibitions, and also gives examples of case notes and patient photographs.

British Red Cross Museum and Archives, London – the history of this organisation in peace and war since 1870, with a valuable research archive; www.redcross.org.uk/museumandarchives.

George Marshall Medical Museum, Worcester – housed on the site of Worcester Royal Hospital, this museum focuses on the evolution of healthcare over the last 250 years; www.medicalmuseum.org.uk.

Glenside Hospital Museum, Bristol – this collection focuses on the history of British psychiatric hospitals and learning disability hospitals; www.glensidemuseum.org.uk.

Hall's Croft, Stratford-upon-Avon – the home of a seventeenth-century physician and displays related to herbal treatments of the period; www.shakespeare.org.uk.

Hunterian Museum, Glasgow – this museum's broad-ranging collection includes the anatomical collection of Dr William Hunter and medical instruments; www.gla.ac.uk/hunterian/collections/.

Hunterian Museum, London – one of Britain's oldest collections of anatomical and pathological specimens based on that of eighteenth-century surgeon John Hunter; www.rcseng.ac.uk.

Museum of Mental Health, Fieldhead Hospital, Ouchthorpe Lane, Wakefield WF1 3SP – tells the story of West Riding Pauper Lunatic Asylum (built 1818). Includes restraining equipment, a padded cell, photographs, and medical equipment. Phone 01924 328654 before visiting.

Old Operating Theatre, London – a beautifully preserved operating theatre from the early nineteenth century and an eighteenth-century garret where apothecaries stored their herbs; www.thegarret.org.uk.

Royal Pharmaceutical Society Museum, London – dedicated to the history of medicines and the profession of pharmacy; www.rpharms.com/about-pharmacy/our-museum.asp.

Royal Victoria Country Park, Southampton – formerly the largest military hospital in the world, but now only the chapel remains which houses a military medicine exhibition; http://www3.hants.gov.uk/rvcp.

Surgeons' Hall Museums, Edinburgh – based at the Royal College of Surgeons, this museum focuses on the history of surgery and dentistry; www.museum.rcsed.ac.uk.

Tayside Medical History Museum, Dundee – located at Ninewells Hospital and Medical School, this is one of the most impressive collections in Scotland; www.dundee.ac.uk/museum.

Thackray Museum, Leeds – a former workhouse on the site of St James's Hospital, it tells the story of medicine and has a valuable archive and library; www.thackraymuseum.org.

Wellcome Collection and Library – this world-famous museum and library is dedicated to the history of health and the human body; the website offers many valuable history resources too; www.wellcomecollection.org.

Welsh Museum of Health and Medicine, Cardiff – a small museum looking at the history of Welsh healthcare; www.wmhm.org.uk.

Worshipful Society of Apothecaries, London – these impressive buildings date from the late 1660s and externally have changed little since that time; www.apothecaries.org.

Other Attractions

This book covers many themes and space precludes a comprehensive listing of all potentially relevant museums and heritage sites. However, here are a few that may be of particular interest:

The Big Pit, Blaenafon, Wales – a chance to tour a real underground coal mine, together with the colliery buildings and medical centre; includes details of mining disasters; www.museumwales.ac.uk/en/bigpit/.

Clink Prison Museum, London – insight into prison life in the past, on the site of the original 'Clink' prison which dated back to the twelfth century; www.clink.co.uk/.

Eyam Museum, Derbyshire – this village was famously ravaged by the plague in 1665, and the local museum devotes much attention to plague history; www.eyammuseum.demon.co.uk/.

Imperial War Museums, London, Duxford, and Manchester – five principal sites explore life for the armed forces personnel and civilians in wars, principally from the twentieth century; www.iwm.org.uk/.

London Dungeon – an interactive exploration of some of London's most dark and sinister past including the plague, Great Fire, Jack the Ripper, and executions; www.the-dungeons.co.uk/london/en/index.htm.

National Maritime Museum, Greenwich – looks at Britain's maritime heritage, both civilian and military, and with an associated research archive and library; www.rmg.co.uk.

BIBLIOGRAPHY

Brown, Kevin. *The Pox – The Life and Near Death of a Very Social Disease.* Sutton Publishing, 2006.

Gately, Iain. *Drink: A Cultural History of Alcohol.* Gotham, 2009.

Harvie, David I. *Limeys: The Conquest of Scurvy.* Sutton Publishing, 2005.

Hempel, Sandra. *The Medical Detective: John Snow, Cholera and the Mystery of the Broad Street Pump.* Granta Books, 2006.

Honigsbaum, Mark. *Living with Enza: The Forgotten Story of Britain and the Great Flu Pandemic of 1918.* Palgrave Macmillan, 2008.

Hurt, Raymond. 'Tuberculosis sanatorium regimen in the 1940s: a patient's personal diary', *Journal of Royal Society of Medicine*, 2004, www.ncbi.nlm.nih.gov/pmc/articles/PMC1079536/.

Loudon, Irvine. *Death in Childbirth: An International Study of Maternal Care and Maternal Mortality 1800–1950.* Clarendon Press, 1992.

Olson, James Stuart. *The History of Cancer: An Annotated Bibliography.* Greenwood Press, 1989.

Porter, Roy. *The Cambridge History of Medicine.* Cambridge University Press, 2006.

Porter, Roy. *The Greatest Benefit to Mankind: A Medical History of Humanity.* Fontana Press, 1999.

Rocco, Fiammetta. *The Miraculous Fever-Tree: Malaria, Medicine, and the Cure that Changed the World.* Harper Collins, 2003.

Scull, Andrew. *The Most Solitary of Afflictions: Madness and Society in Britain 1700–1900.* Yale University Press, 1993.

Shaw, Anne and Reeves, Carole. *The Children of Craig-y-nos: Life in a Welsh Tuberculosis Sanatorium, 1922–1959.* Wellcome Trust, 2009.

Shrewsbury, JFD. *A History of Bubonic Plague in the British Isles.* Cambridge University Press, 1970.

Talty, Stephen. *The Illustrious Dead: The Terrifying Story of How Typhus Killed Napoleon's Greatest Army.* Three Rivers Press, 2010.

Webb, Simon. *Execution: A History of Capital Punishment in Britain.* The History Press, 2011.

INDEX

abdominal typhus, *see* typhoid
abortion, 147–8
abruption, 145
accidental haemorrhage, 149
accidents, 4, 25, 30–9, 45
African sleeping sickness, 168
ague, 168
alcohol/alcoholism, 29, 40–6
American plague, *see* yellow fever
amputation, 198–200
aneurysm, 96
angina, 113–14, 115
animals as medicines, *see* medicines
anthrax, 58–9
antiscorbutics, *see* scurvy
apoplexy, 95, 96–8, 114
apothecaries, 15, 208
appendicitis, 1, 92–3
army fever, *see* typhus
arrhythmia, 96
artificial limbs, 199
aspirin, 14
asthma, 2, 53–5, 57, 111
asylums, 16, 119–23, 126–9

baby, definition by age, 61
behaviour, and disease, 6
beheading, 101
bilharzia, 168
Black Assizes, 180–1
Black Death, *see* plague
blacklegs, *see* scurvy
black vomit, *see* yellow fever
blackwater fever, *see* malaria
bleeding a patient (bloodletting), 8
bleeding and childbirth, *see*
    childbirth, death in

blistering, as treatment, 9
blood poisoning, 200
Bloody Assizes, 195
bloody flux, *see* dysentery
blue plague, *see* cholera
bombing, 195
botulism, 84–5
bronchitis, 2, 53, 57, 59
bronze John, *see* yellow fever
buboes, 138, 183
bubonic plague, *see* plague
burned at the stake, 101–2

calomel, *see* mercury as medicine
camp fever, *see* typhus
campaign fever, *see* dysentery
cancer, 1, 2, 47–52, 56
capital punishment, *see* execution
carcinoma, *see* cancer
catarrhal fever, *see* influenza
cathartics, *see* laxatives
cemeteries, 24, 203–5
cerebral haemorrhage, 97
cerebrovascular accident, *see* stroke
charbon, *see* anthrax
chemotherapy, 48–9, 50
chest diseases, 53–60
chest infection, 2, 53, 59
child, definition by age, 61
childbed fever, 148
childbirth, death in, 143–9, 201
childhood deaths, 31, 61–99, *see also*
    life expectancy
chink cough, *see* whooping cough
cholera, 4, 11, 70–6, 204, 205
cholera morbus, 75
cholera nostras, 75

chrisome, 62
Christianity, *see* Church and
    healing
Church and healing, 14, 15
clap, the, *see* venereal disease
clinical trials, 6–7, 11
clysters, 8
coalmining, 30, 57–8, 59, 208
congenital syphilis, 186
congestive fever, *see* malaria
consumption, *see* tuberculosis (TB)
convulsions, 2, 69, 95–6
coronary thrombosis, *see* heart
    attack
coroners' inquests, 21, 25
corruption, 198
court proceedings, *see* legal sources
    about deaths
courts martial, 99, 193
cretin, 84, 130
criminal trials, *see* legal sources
    about deaths
croops, *see* croup
croup, 68–9
Cupid's disease, *see* venereal
    disease
cupping, 9
curse of Venus, *see* venereal disease
cynanche parotidea, *see* mumps

death certificates, 17–19
death sentence, *see* execution
deaths abroad, 19, 25
debility, 18
deep-vein thrombosis, 149
dementia, 2, 130
dengue fever, 168
Derbyshire Neck, 84
despondency, 130
Devonshire colic, 85
diagnosis, 1–7
diet, and disease, 6
diphtheria, 4, 62–4
disasters, *see* accidents
disease, theories 5–6
dock fever, *see* yellow fever
doctors, 15
Doctrine of Signatures, 9
dropsy, *see* heart failure
drowning, 32–3, *see also* shipwrecks

drunkenness, *see*
    alcohol/alcoholism
Dutch distemper, *see* scurvy
dysentery, 4, 86–91, 168
dyspnoea, 111

eclampsia, 148
eclamptic fits, 148
effusion on brain, *see* stroke
elder decline, 18
emetics, 8
emphysema, 59
endometritis, 148
enemas, 8
enteric fever, *see* typhoid
environment, and disease, 6
epidemic, 29
epidemic catarrh, *see* influenza
epilepsy, 94–6, *see also* convulsions
ergotism, 85
erysipelas, 201
execution
    by armed forces, 99, 193–4
    by State, 99–108, 195
exhaustion of vital powers, 18, 130

falling sickness, *see* epilepsy
falls, 33–4
famine, *see* starvation
feeble-minded, 130
fever, 1, 69, 148, 165
'fever islands', 164
feveret, *see* influenza
filariasis, 168
fires, 33
firing squad, 194
fits, *see* convulsions, epilepsy
flogging to death, 194
flu, *see* influenza
flux, *see* dysentery
foreign death certificates, 19
foundry workers, 57
French Pox, 184

gangrene, 198–9
gaol fever/distemper, *see* typhus
gassing, in wartime, 192–3
gastric fever, *see* typhoid
general paralysis of the insane, 183
German measles, *see* rubella

gibbeting, 100
gonorrhoea, *see* venereal disease
gravestones, *see* memorials
Great Plague of London, *see* plague
Great Pox, 183
griping in the guts, 1, 91–3
grippe, *see* influenza
gummata, 183

haemorrhage and childbirth, *see* childbirth, death in
haemorrhagic fever, *see* yellow fever
hanging
    in chains, 100
    as State execution, 99–108
    of self, *see* suicide
    from yardarm, 194
headstones, *see* memorials
heart attack, 96, 114–15
heart disease, 2, 109–15
heart failure, 1, 111–13
hepatitis, 52
herbs as medicines, *see* medicines
hospital fever, *see* typhus
hospitals, 15, 26–7, 206–7
humoural theory, 5
humours, 5
hypertensive disease of pregnancy, 148
hysteria, 130

idiot, meaning of, 127
imbecile, meaning of, 127, 130
immunisation, *see* vaccination
infant, definition by age, 61
infantile paralysis, *see* polio
influenza, 2, 116–18
inoculation, *see* vaccination
ipecacuanha, 8
inquests, *see* coroner

jail fever, *see* typhus
jaundice, 52
journals, 20, 29

Kassowitz's law, 186
king's evil, 175
knife grinders, 57
Koch's disease, *see* tuberculosis (TB)

laudanum, 133
laxatives, 8
lead poisoning, 85
leather industry, 58
leeches, *see* bleeding a patient
legal sources about deaths, 21–2, 25, 105–6
leishmaniasis, 168
leprosy, 167
leptospirosis, 52
life expectancy, 4
lockjaw, *see* tetanus
lunacy, *see* mental illness
lunatic, meaning of, 127
lupus vulgaris, 175

madhouses, *see* asylums
magazines, 20
malaria, 14, 166–8
malignancy, *see* cancer
malignant sore throat, *see* diphtheria
malnutrition, 4, 79, *see also* starvation
malthouses, 57
mania, 130
marasmus, 83
marsh fever, *see* malaria
marsh miasm, *see* malaria
measles, 64
medicines, 9–14, 48
melancholia, 130
membranous croup, *see* diphtheria
memorials, 23–4, 203–5
meningitis, 2, 64–5
mental illness, 119–30, 206–7
    after pregnancy, 146, 149
mercury as medicine, 10–11, 187
metals as medicines, *see* medicines
metastases/metastatic, *see* cancer
metria, 148
miasma, 73, 166
midwives, 15
milk leg, 149
mill-workers, 57
minerals as medicines, *see* medicines
mining accidents, *see* coalmining
monasteries, *see* Church and healing

mongolism, 130
morbilli, *see* measles
morphine, 14
mortification, 198
mumps, 65
murder, 21, 99–108
museums, health-related, 206–7
mustard plasters, 9
myocardial infarction, *see* heart attack

National Burial Index, 24
natural decay, 18, 130
neonate, 61
nerves, 130
nervous fever, *see* typhoid
newspapers, 20, 24–6, 106, 195
nostrums, 12
nurses, 15

obituaries, 20
occupational deaths, 30–6, 57–9
old age, 2, 4, 18, 31
old-age decline, 130
onchocerciasis, 168
opium, 14, 131–7
opium overdose, 136
osteomalacia, 84

palsy, 96
paludal poison, *see* malaria
paralysis, 18, 96
    of the insane, 183
paregoric, 133
paresis, 96
parish records, 22–3
parotitis, *see* mumps
patent medicines, 12–13
pellagra, 84
pelvic abscess, 148
peptic ulcer, *see* ulcer, of bowel
peritonitis, 92, 93, 144
pertussis, *see* whooping cough
pestilential fever, 181
petechial fever, *see* typhus
pharmacists, 15
phlegmasia dolens, 149
phthisis, *see* tuberculosis
physicians, 15
placenta praevia, 145

placental abruption, 149
plague, 2, 138–42, 204, 208
plane crash, 37
plant medicines, *see* medicines
pleurisy/pleuritis, 2, 60
pneumonia, *see* chest infection
poisoning
    by self, *see* suicide
    via food, 84–5
polio/poliomyelitis, 66
Poor Law unions, *see* workhouses
postnatal diseases, 148–9
postpartum diseases, 148–9
potato famines, 80–1
Pott's disease, 175
pre-eclampsia, 148
pregnancy, death in, *see* childbirth, death in
prison fever, *see* typhus
psychiatric illness, *see* mental illness
puerperal diseases, 146–7
puerperal fever, 143–9, 201
pulmonary embolism, 96, 149
purgatives, *see* laxatives
purpura nautica, *see* scurvy
purulence, 200
purulent fever, 200
putrefaction, 198
putrid fever, *see* diphtheria or typhus
pyaemia, 200
pythogenic fever, *see* typhoid

quartan fever, 168
quinine, 14, 167

rachitis, *see* rickets
radiotherapy, 48, 51
railway accidents, 25, 36–7
relapsing fever, 168
remittent fever, infantile, *see* typhoid
remitting fever, *see* malaria
retained placenta and flooding, 149
rheumatic fever, 67–8, 112
rickets, 84, 146
river blindness, 168
road accidents, 36–7
rubella, 66
rubeola, *see* measles
St Anthony's fire, 85

sanitation, 4, *see also* cholera, dysentery
scarlatina, *see* scarlet fever
scarlet fever, 67–8, 201
schistosomiasis, 168
scirrhus, *see* cancer
scorbie/scorbutus, *see* scurvy
scrofula, 175
scurvy, 11, 150–6
sea, deaths at, *see* drowning, shipwrecks
seizures, *see* convulsions, epilepsy, stroke
senility, 18, 130
sepsis, 200–1
septicaemia, 200
setons, 9
sewage, *see* sanitation
shell shock, 130
ship's fever, *see* typhus
shipwrecks, 34–6
sinapisms, 9
smallpox, 2, 4, 11, 61, 157–63
smoking, *see* tobacco
social diseases, *see* venereal disease
sphacelus, 198
splenic fever, *see* anthrax
spotted fever, *see* typhus
starvation, 77–84, 194
stillbirth/stillborn, 61, 186
stonemasons, 57
stranger's fever, *see* yellow fever
stroke, 2, 94–8
sudden death, 96, 114, 149
suffocative catarrh, 111
suicide, 124–6
suppuration, 198
suppurative fever, 200
surgeons/surgery, 15, 47, 50, 197, 199, 207
swamp sickness, *see* malaria
sweating sickness, 2
syphilis, *see* venereal disease
syphilis, congenital, 186

tabes mesenterica, 175
tetanus, 201–2
thyroid, 84
tissick, 53, 175
tobacco, 54, 55–7

toxaemia of pregnancy, 145–6
treatments, for disease, 6–14
trench fever, 192
trench foot, 192
trials, criminal, *see* legal sources about deaths
trismus, 202
trypanosomiasis, 168
tuberculosis (TB), 2, 4, 53, 169–75
tumour, *see* cancer
tussis convulsiva, *see* whooping cough
typhoid, 4, 89–91, 201
typhus, 2, 4, 176–82

ulcer
of bowel, 1, 92
of skin, 198
unsound mind, 130

vaccination, 4, 61–9, 90–1, 119, 159–62, 166, 174, 180, 202
vapours, the, 130
varicella, 159
variola, *see* smallpox
venereal disease, 183–9
violence, *see* accidents, murder, war, death in
vitamin A poisoning, 85
vitamin deficiencies, 84

war, death in, 190–5, 205, 208
weakness, 96
weather, and disease/death, 6, 31
Weil's disease, 52
white man's grave, 164
white plague, *see* tuberculosis
whooping cough, 2, 68–9
womb fever, 148
wool-sorter's disease, *see* anthrax
workhouses, 16, 27–8, 82–3, 120, 129–30, 207
wounds, 196–202

X-rays, 48

yaws, 168
yellow fever, 164–6, 168
yellow jack, *see* yellow fever
youth, definition by age, 61

Read all about it! World's largest collection of local British newspapers now available at findmypast.co.uk!

Learn about your ancestors' lives over the last 250 years...

With the British newspaper collection

- Uncover fascinating stories about your very own ancestors in over 6 million local British newspaper pages from the British Library - the collection is growing every day
- Find out what happened down your street 100 years ago
- Read the headlines and articles just as your ancestors read them throughout their lives
- Understand the key events that shaped your family's lives

Claim 20 free credits at findmypast.co.uk/ancestors now!

Terms & conditions apply. See website for details.

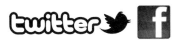

Twitter: **findmypast**   Facebook: **findmypast UK**

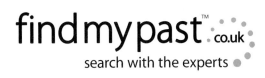

search with the experts